Techniques in Facial Plastic Surgery: Discussion and Debate

Guest Editors

FRED G. FEDOK, MD
ROBERT M. KELLMAN, MD

FACIAL PLASTIC SURGERY CLINICS OF NORTH AMERICA

www.facialplastic.theclinics.com

Consulting Editor
J. REGAN THOMAS, MD, FACS

August 2012 • Volume 20 • Number 3

SAUNDERS an imprint of ELSEVIER, Inc.

W.B. SAUNDERS COMPANY
A Division of Elsevier Inc.

1600 John F. Kennedy Blvd., Suite 1800, Philadelphia, PA 19103-2899

http://www.theclinics.com

FACIAL PLASTIC SURGERY CLINICS OF NORTH AMERICA Volume 20, Number 3
August 2012 ISSN 1064-7406, ISBN 978-1-4557-3859-5

Editor: Joanne Husovski

Facial Plastic Surgery Clinics of North America (ISSN 1064-7406) is published quarterly by Elsevier Inc., 360 Park Avenue South, New York, NY 10010-1710. Months of issue are February, May, August, and November. Business and Editorial Offices: 1600 John F. Kennedy Blvd., Suite 1800, Philadelphia, PA 19103-2899. Periodicals postage paid at New York, NY, and additional mailing offices. Subscription prices are $359.00 per year (US individuals), $496.00 per year (US institutions), $409.00 per year (Canadian individuals), $594.00 per year (Canadian institutions), $489.00 per year (foreign individuals), $594.00 per year (foreign institutions), $170.00 per year (US students), and $237.00 per year (foreign students). Foreign air speed delivery is included in all *Clinics* subscription prices. All prices are subject to change without notice. POSTMASTER: Send address changes to *Facial Plastic Surgery Clinics*, Elsevier Health Sciences Division, Subscription Customer Service, 3251 Riverport Lane, Maryland Heights, MO 63043. **Customer service: 1-800-654-2452 (US and Canada); 1-314-447-8871 (outside US and Canada); Fax: 314-447-8029; E-mail:journalscustomerservice-usa@elsevier.com (for print support); journalsonlinesupport-usa@elsevier.com (for online support).**

Reprints. For copies of 100 or more of articles in this publication, please contact the Commercial Reprints Department, Elsevier Inc., 360 Park Avenue South, New York, NY 10010-1710. Tel.: 212-633-3812; Fax: 212-462-1935; E-mail: reprints@elsevier.com.

Facial Plastic Surgery Clinics of North America is covered in *MEDLINE/PubMed* (*Index Medicus*).

Printed and bound by CPI Group (UK) Ltd, Croydon, CR0 4YY

Transferred to Digital Print 2012

Contributors

CONSULTING EDITOR

J. REGAN THOMAS, MD, FACS
Professor and Chairman, Department of
Otolaryngology, University of Illinois at
Chicago, Chicago, Illinois

GUEST EDITORS

FRED G. FEDOK, MD, FACS
Professor and Chief, Facial Plastic and
Reconstructive Surgery, Otolaryngology/
Head and Neck Surgery, Department of
Surgery, The Hershey Medical Center,
The Pennsylvania State University,
Hershey, Pennsylvania

ROBERT M. KELLMAN, MD
President-elect, American Academy of Facial
Plastic & Reconstructive Surgery, Professor
and Chair, Department of Otolaryngology and
Communication Sciences, State University of
New York–Upstate Medical University,
Syracuse, New York

AUTHORS

ONEIDA AROSARENA, MD
Associate Professor, Department of
Otolaryngology–Head and Neck Surgery,
Temple University, Philadelphia, Pennsylvania

KOFI BOAHENE, MD
Assistant Professor of Facial Plastic and
Reconstructive Surgery, Department of
Otolaryngology–Head and Neck Surgery,
Johns Hopkins University School of Medicine,
Baltimore, Maryland

PATRICK BYRNE, MD
Associate Professor and Director of Facial
Plastic and Reconstructive Surgery,
Department of Otolaryngology–Head and Neck
Surgery; Fellowship Director, Facial Plastic and
Reconstructive Surgery, Johns Hopkins
University School of Medicine, Baltimore,
Maryland

STEVEN H. DAYAN, MD, FACS
Chicago Center for Facial Plastic Surgery;
Assistant Professor of Otolaryngology, Division
of Facial Plastic Surgery, Department of
Otolaryngology, University of Illinois at
Chicago; Adjunct Professor, School of New
Learning, DePaul University, Chicago, Illinois

YADRANKO DUCIC, MD, FRCS(C), FACS
Clinical Professor, Department of
Otolaryngology–Head and Neck Surgery,
University of Texas Southwestern Medical
Center, Dallas; Codirector, Baylor
Neuroscience Center Skullbase Program;
Otolaryngology and Facial Plastic Surgery
Associates, Fort Worth, Texas

DAVID A.F. ELLIS, MD, FRCSC
Professor, Division of Facial Plastic Surgery,
Department of Otolaryngology–Head and Neck
Surgery, University of Toronto; Medical
Director, Art of Facial Surgery, Toronto,
Ontario, Canada

EDWARD ELLIS III, DDS, MS
Chair and Professor, Department of Oral and
Maxillofacial Surgery, The University of Texas
Health Science Center at San Antonio,
San Antonio, Texas

MARK GLASGOLD, MD
Glasgold Group Plastic Surgery, Highland
Park, New Jersey

ROBERT M. KELLMAN, MD
President-elect, American Academy of Facial Plastic & Reconstructive Surgery, Professor and Chair, Department of Otolaryngology and Communication Sciences, State University of New York – Upstate Medical University, Syracuse, New York

SAMUEL LAM, MD
Lam Facial Plastic Surgery Center, Plano, Texas

BRIAN P. MALONEY, MD
Maloney Center for Facial Plastic Surgery, Atlanta, Georgia

E. GAYLON MCCOLLOUGH, MD
McCollough Plastic Surgery Clinic, Gulf Shores, Alabama

MARY LYNN MORAN, MD
Facial Plastic and Reconstructive Surgery, Woodside, California

STEPHEN PERKINS, MD
Meridian Plastic Surgeons, Indianapolis, Indiana

BARRY M. SCHAITKIN, MD
Professor, Department of Otolaryngology, University of Pittsburgh, Pittsburgh, Pennsylvania

J. REGAN THOMAS, MD
Professor and Chairman, Department of Otolaryngology, University of Illinois at Chicago, Chicago, Illinois

TRAVIS T. TOLLEFSON, MD, MPH
Cleft and Craniofacial Program, Otolaryngology–Head and Neck Surgery, Associate Professor, Facial Plastic and Reconstructive Surgery, University of California, Davis, Sacramento, California

WILLIAM TRUSWELL IV, MD
Clinical Instructor, Private Practice, The University of Connecticut School of Medicine; Aesthetic Laser and Cosmetic Surgery Center, Northampton, Massachusetts

THOMAS L. TZIKAS, MD
Facial Plastic Surgeon, Delray Beach, Florida

S. RANDOLPH WALDMAN, MD
Waldman Plastic Surgery Center, Lexington, Kentucky

EMRE VURAL, MD
Associate Professor, Department of Otolaryngology–Head and Neck Surgery, University of Arkansas for Medical Sciences, Little Rock, Arkansas

Contents

Brian P. Maloney, William Truswell IV, and S. Randolph Waldman address questions for discussion and debate:

1. Is surgery ever a better alternative than injectable fillers for enhancement of the lips?

2. What role do permanent lip implants play for today's patients?

3. How do you manage the small mouth person seeking lip enlargement?

4. How do you handle down-turning corners of the mouth?

5. How do you handle a person who previously had full lips but now is losing volume, especially in the corners?

6. What qualities of the lip are important to preserve when considering various lip augmentation materials and techniques?

7. What are the best ways of reducing the length of the upper lip?

8. Analysis: Over the past 5 years, how has your technique or approach to lips changed, or what is the most important thing you have learned in performing lip augmentations.

Oneida Arosarena, Yadranko Ducic, and Travis T. Tollefson address questions for discussion and debate:

1. Is rigid fixation essential for the treatment of angle fractures, or is a single plate along the superior border sufficient?

2. Does the presence of teeth in the fracture line (particularly the third molar in angle fractures) contribute to stability of the fixation, or is it a nidus for infection?

3. What is the role of postoperative antibiotics? Are they always necessary?

4. Do you believe that applying MMF is an important part of mandibular fracture repair? If you do not use MMF in all cases, how do you decide which cases require intraoperative and/or postoperative MMF? Do you believe that the techniques/methods of applying MMF make a difference?

5. How do you manage edentulous mandible fractures?

6. Analysis: Over the past 5 years, how has your technique or approach changed or what is the most important thing you have learned in dealing with mandible fractures?

Edward Ellis III, Robert M. Kellman, and Emre Vural address questions for discussion and debate:

1. Are there specific indications for open versus closed treatment of subcondylar fractures? Are there any contraindications to open treatment, and do they supercede the indications for open treatment?

2. Does the presence of other fractures (mandible and/or midface) affect your choice of open versus closed treatment? (Is the selection of closed vs open treatment the same for unilateral vs bilateral fractures?)

3. If one chooses to perform closed treatment, how long a period of MMF is required?

4. What are the most important factors for success when closed treatment is used?

5. What is the best surgical approach to ORIF of subcondylar fractures?

6. Analysis: Over the past 5 years, how has your technique or approach evolved or what is the most important thing you have learned/observed in working with subcondylar fractures?

Kofi Boahene, Patrick Byrne, and Barry M. Schaitkin address questions for discussion and debate:

1. What forms of nonsurgical therapy (physical therapy, electrical stimulation, and so forth) do you recommend to improve the outcome of facial paralysis and why?

2. Explain your preoperative assessment tool for deciding what to do (Eye reanimation? Who needs a medial canthoplasty? and so forth).

3. How do you assess the results of management of facial paralysis?

4. Discuss the use of end-to-side anastomosis (Viterbo concept of something for nothing). Should it be used; why or why not?

5. What is your preferred method for temporalis muscle transposition and why? Are there any tricks to improving the results?

6. Do you use cross-facial nerve jump grafts and use them for free muscle innervation? If so, what are the pearls you have learned from this technique and when do you use it?

7. Analysis: Over the past 5 years, how has your approach evolved or what have you learned/observed in working with reanimation.

Advisory Board to Facial Plastic Surgery Clinics 2012

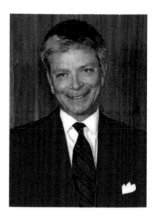
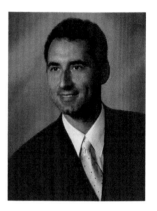
Facial Plastic Surgery Clinics is pleased to introduce the 2012 **Advisory Board**.

Facial Plastic Surgery Clinics is widely available through the media of print, digital e-Reader, online via the Internet, and on iPad and smart phones.

Facial Plastic Surgery Clinics provides professionals access to pertinent point-of-care answers and current clinical information, along with comprehensive background information for deeper understanding.

Readers are welcome to contact the Clinics Editor or Board with comments.

BOARD MEMBERS 2012

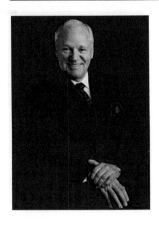
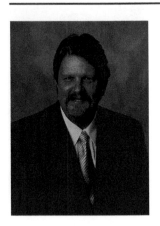
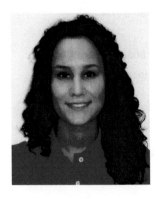

STEVEN FAGIEN, MD, FACS

Aesthetic Eyelid Plastic Surgery
660 Glades Road; Suite 210
Boca Raton, Florida 33431

561.393.9898
sfagien@aol.com

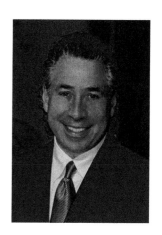

GREG KELLER, MD

Clinical Professor of Surgery, Head and Neck,
David Geffen School of Medicine,
University of California, Los Angeles;

Keller Facial Plastic Surgery
221 W. Pueblo St. Ste A
Santa Barbara, CA 93105

805.687.6408
faclft@aol.com
www.gregorykeller.com

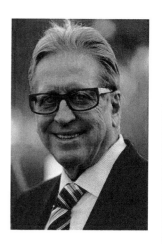

THEDA C. KONTIS, MD

Assistant Professor, Johns Hopkins Hospital
Facial Plastic Surgicenter, Ltd.
1838 Greene Tree Road, Suite 370
Baltimore, MD 21208

410.486.3400
tckontis@aol.com
www.facialplasticsurgerymd.com
www.facial-plasticsurgery.com

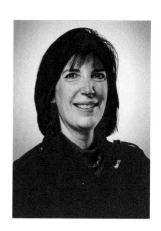

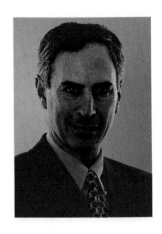

IRA D. PAPEL, MD

Facial Plastic Surgicenter
Associate Professor
The Johns Hopkins University
1838 Greene Tree Road, Suite 370
Baltimore, MD 21208

410.486.3400
idpmd@aol.com
www.facial-plasticsurgery.com

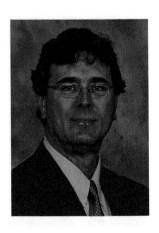

SHERARD A. TATUM, MD

Professor of Otolaryngology and
Pediatrics Cleft and Craniofacial Center
Division of Facial Plastic Surgery
Upstate Medical University
750 E. Adams St.
Syracuse, NY 13210

315.464.4636
TatumS@upstate.edu
www.upstate.edu

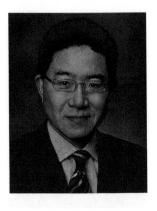

TOM D. WANG, MD

Professor
Facial Plastic and Reconstructive Surgery
Oregon Health & Science University
3181 Southwest Sam Jackson Park Road
Portland, OR 97239

503.494.5678
wangt@ohsu.edu
www.ohsu.edu/drtomwang

FACIAL PLASTIC SURGERY CLINICS OF NORTH AMERICA

FORTHCOMING ISSUES

Non-melanoma Skin Cancer of the Head and Neck
Cemal Cingi, MD, *Guest Editor*

Skin: Essentials for Facial Reconstruction
David Hom, MD, and Adam Ingraffea, MD, *Guest Editors*

Minimally Invasive Procedures in Facial Plastic Surgery
Theda Kontis, MD, *Guest Editor*

RECENT ISSUES

May 2012
Emerging Tools and Trends in Facial Plastic Surgery
Paul J. Carniol, MD, *Guest Editor*

February 2012
Rhinology and Allergy for the Facial Plastic Surgeon
Stephanie A. Joe, MD, *Guest Editor*

November 2011
3D Imaging Technologies for Facial Plastic Surgery
John Pallanch, MD, MS, *Guest Editor*

Foreword
Facial Plastic Surgery Clinics "Debate" Issue

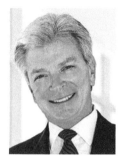

J. Regan Thomas, MD
Consulting Editor

Facial plastic surgery continues on a path of rapid growth and development both in the technology utilized in facial plastic surgery as well as in the evolution of surgical technique. *Facial Plastic Surgery Clinics* continues to be a well-respected source of information for both the experienced practicing facial plastic surgeon as well as the individuals in various levels of their training programs. This is accomplished by providing an up-to-date and current resource contributed by active experts in the field as guest editors who with contributions of their invited authors demonstrate appropriate steps to provide the best facial plastic surgery outcomes for patients based on their expertise and experience. The contributions of these authors collectively then make training and experience possible from a variety of medical specialties, all of which provide a valuable fund of knowledge. *Facial Plastic Surgery Clinics* is a key educational source for the field and is always looking for new and innovative ways to provide insight as well as knowledge in the realm of this expanding specialty.

Through discussion with the *Facial Plastic Surgery Clinics* Editorial Board it was felt that a comparative discussion of technique and experience by expert surgeons and contributors would be useful on a specific topic-based approach. The concept was, for a variety of given specific topics, that those individual experts would discuss their perspective and even be given the latitude and encouragement to debate areas of disagreement. In this way the reader would be able to benefit from that diversity of opinion and surgical approach. Drs Bob Kellman

and Fred Fedok, both respected facial plastic surgery experts in their own right, were asked to lead this project as our guest editors. This is the first in a series in *Facial Plastic Surgery Clinic* issues where Drs Kellman and Fedok developed an intriguing approach to pose 5 different questions to each guest author for response. This would then allow discussions from these experienced surgeons as to their technique, their rationale, and their experience. They would be encouraged to discuss their own evolution of thought in these techniques, which had been developed over time. The authors likewise were encouraged to provide technique videos for appropriate cases, and the reader will have access through *Facial Plastic Surgery Clinic* to view these as well. The reader should be able to utilize this to augment and combine the experience and opinions of the "Masters" with the readers' own approach to their patients. The *Facial Plastic Surgery Clinics* is delighted to provide this intriguing and educational approach to its readership. It will no doubt become an important component of the facial plastic surgeon's personal library.

J. Regan Thomas, MD
Department of Otolaryngology–
Head and Neck Surgery
University of Illinois, Chicago
1855 West Taylor Street, MC 648
Chicago, IL 60612, USA

E-mail address:
thomasrj@uic.edu

Facial Plast Surg Clin N Am 20 (2012) xv
http://dx.doi.org/10.1016/j.fsc.2012.07.001
1064-7406/12/$ – see front matter © 2012 Elsevier Inc. All rights reserved.

facialplastic.theclinics.com

Preface
Facial Plastic Surgery: Discussion and Debate

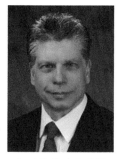 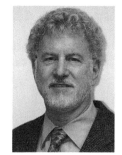

Fred G. Fedok, MD   Robert M. Kellman, MD
Guest Editors

An expert, by definition, is one "...whose special knowledge or skill causes him to be regarded as an authority; a specialist" (Oxford English Dictionary). When well-educated, highly experienced experts get together and express their opinions, very interesting things happen: ... *learning grows* from compound experience and education; *disagreements are voiced* as each expert advocates for their view; *insights are gained* from fine shades of difference; and *everyone observing comes away better off* for having been in the company of experts.

In this issue of *Facial Plastic Surgery Clinics*, invited expert surgeons in the field of cosmetic and reconstructive facial surgery come together to form panels to discuss 6 questions on procedural approaches for facelift, facial fillers, chemical peels, fat grafting, lip augmentation, mandible fractures, subcondylar fractures, and facial reanimation. The questions vary to best address frequently controversial and debated issues about the procedure under discussion, but common to every discussion is the same question asked of each expert: *What have you learned or how has your approach changed over the past few years and why*? This 1 question alone provides readers a glimpse into the evolution of thought, technique, and expertise of the finest facial plastic surgeons practicing today.

The rapid and dramatic stretching of limits in science and technology and technique is pushing this field to artfully perform techniques not possible just a decade ago. The veritable explosion of "cosmetic experts" and techniques has put into the reach and into the consciousness of the general public the potential for plastic surgery formerly available to only a small population. In reflecting the highly individualized nature of Facial Plastic Surgery, we chose this innovative publication format to provide an interplay of responses between experts much like a live panel. The goal of each article is to allow the panelists to discuss "issues" and offer their personal thoughts—particularly the opportunity to compare and contrast with the ideas of other experts—about a technique and treatment, rather than to have the article narrowly focus on only 1 author's experience. As we continue to educate ourselves in the best techniques and methods available to provide the best outcomes, we all continue to grow from listening to one another and challenging our own methods in this artistic specialty.

This is volume 1 of a 2-volume panel discussion and debate among experts. Interestingly, we as guest editors found ourselves learning and growing merely from determining which were the most important questions; we sincerely hope that our fellow surgeons and surgeons-in-training come away with minds wide open and enthusiasm to continue

Facial Plast Surg Clin N Am 20 (2012) xvii–xviii
http://dx.doi.org/10.1016/j.fsc.2012.07.002

facialplastic.theclinics.com

evolving with the best techniques available after reading this issue. Read on and enjoy!

Fred G. Fedok, MD
Facial Plastic and Reconstructive Surgery
Otolaryngology/Head and Neck Surgery
Department of Surgery
The Hershey Medical Center
The Pennsylvania State University
500 University Drive
Hershey, PA 17033, USA

Robert M. Kellman, MD
Department of Otolaryngology and
Communication Sciences
State University of New York –
Upstate Medical University
750 East Adams Street
Syracuse, NY 13210, USA

E-mail addresses:
ffedok@hmc.psu.edu (F.G. Fedok)
kellmanr@upstate.edu (R.M. Kellman)

Facial Fillers: Discussion and Debate

Steven H. Dayan, MD[a,b,c,*], David A.F. Ellis, MD, FRCSC[d,e,*],
Mary Lynn Moran, MD[f,*]

KEYWORDS

- Facial fillers • Collagen injection • Anesthesia • Panel discussion

---

Facial Fillers Panel Discussion

Steven H. Dayan, David Ellis, and Mary Lynn Moran address questions about facial fillers for discussion and debate:

1. Are there different indications for the different fillers?
2. In your opinion, what are the durations of the various fillers?
3. Is there still a role for the use of collagen injections?
4. What complications concern you and what do you do in your practice to attempt to avoid or minimize these?
5. What type of anesthesia do you use, when, and why?
6. *Analysis:* Over the past 5 years, how have you modified your techniques or approach or what is the most important thing you have learned/observed in working with injectables and fillers?

 Dr Dayan presents a video of his technique for facial fillers using a blunt tip cannula. Available at: http://www.facialplastic.theclinics.com/

Are there different indications for the different fillers?

DAYAN

It has been my impression that, as we gain more experience, the greater are the apparent differences between the various fillers approved by the Food and Drug Administration (FDA). Once recognized, each filler's unique physical properties can be relied on to achieve specific outcomes in individual patients. Furthermore, the fillers are priced differently, have different durations, and are marketed differently. All of these factors ought to be taken into consideration before deciding which filler is best for a patient.

Hyaluronic acid fillers

The most popular fillers are the hyaluronic acids (HAs), as they comprised 85% (1.3 million of the 1.5 million) of the filler treatments in 2010.[1]

The 2 leading brands Restylane/Perlane (Medicis Aesthetics, Scottsdale, AZ, USA) and Juvéderm Ultra/Ultraplus (Allergan, Irvine, CA, USA) make

---

[a] Chicago Center for Facial Plastic Surgery, 845 North Michigan Avenue, Suite 923 East, Chicago, IL 60611, USA
[b] Division of Facial Plastic Surgery, Department of Otolaryngology, University of Illinois at Chicago, Chicago, IL, USA
[c] School of New Learning, DePaul University, Chicago, IL, USA
[d] Division of Facial Plastic Surgery, Department of Otolaryngology–Head and Neck Surgery, University of Toronto, Toronto, Ontario, Canada
[e] Art of Facial Surgery, 167 Sheppard Avenue West, Toronto, Ontario M2N 1M9, Canada
[f] Facial Plastic and Reconstructive Surgery, 2973 Woodside Road, Woodside, CA 94062, USA
* Corresponding authors.
E-mail addresses: sdayan@drdayan.com; ellis2106@gmail.com; mlmoranmd@yahoo.com

Facial Plast Surg Clin N Am 20 (2012) 245–264
doi:10.1016/j.fsc.2012.05.004
1064-7406/12/$ – see front matter © 2012 Elsevier Inc. All rights reserved.

up most of the market share, and although they are often thought of interchangeably they have very different physical properties.[2] Juvéderm is positioned as the "smoother filler." Its gel-like 24 mg/mL concentration with hydrophilic properties 6 times that of Restylane is likely the reason behind its smoother effects.[3] Restylane, a firmer product defined by its rheological properties G',[3] is more than 6 times more resistant than Juvéderm to deformation.

It is these precise differences between Juvéderm and Restylane that I frequently rely on for specific indications. Juvéderm-corrected areas tend to lead to a fuller and more diffuse augmentation as water is absorbed. I also have noticed that the Juvéderm augmentation may be dynamically related to the body's current levels of hydration. Anecdotally I have a young staff member who, after receiving Juvéderm into her lips, has a noticeably variable augmentation of her lips the day after she has a meal of salty food. I have not witnessed this with the less hydrophilic Restylane. Consequently, knowledge of its greater hydrophilicity can be used to an advantage, especially in the lips (**Fig. 1**). For the younger patient who is seeking enlarged lips and already has a full body lip, I will place 0.4 mL of Juvéderm deep into each lip body. For the more mature patient with natively thinner lips and/or who is overly concerned about a recognizable difference, I will place a fine whisper (0.3–0.5 mL) of Restylane within either vermilion border. This procedure has the effect of obviating fine vertical rhytids of the lip and nicely defining the lip border without extending into the cutaneous lip or body. Lipstick can now be placed without concerns of migration, and the lips appear more youthful but not enlarged.

However, because of its firmer nature and less hydrophilic properties, Restylane can lead to lumps and irregularities if not placed evenly. Juvéderm, with its highly hydrophilic nature, tends to attract more fluid and, therefore, results in a diffuse filling effect, which I believe with its nonparticulate gel consistency work to deliver its marketed "smoother" effect. However, if a larger quantity of Juvéderm (more than 1.0 mL approximately) is placed into a lip, it can rather quickly lead to an unnatural, large shelf-like appearance of the cutaneous white lip.

Beyond the lips, the differences in hydrophilic nature of the HAs can also be relied on when correcting or augmenting the nasolabial folds (NLF) and cheeks. For the buccal cheek space, I find Juvéderm's superior hydrophilic and diffuse filling

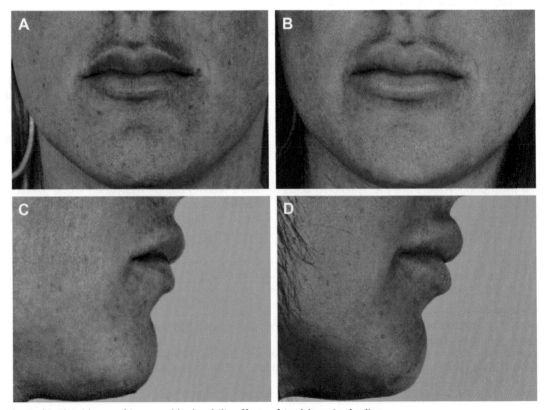

Fig. 1. (*A–D*) Evidence of increased hydrophilic effects of Juvéderm in the lips.

properties more beneficial, whereas in the infraorbital tear trough I prefer Restylane. Nowhere on the face are the differences between Juvéderm and Restylane more apparent than when placed into the loose areolar tissues surrounding the orbital region. I find Juvéderm to be contraindicated because it will reliably swell, resulting in dark puffy undereye circles representative of a tired unflattering appearance. Although it can occur with both products under the eyes, the Tyndall effect, whereby optical chamber of HA and fluid reflects blue light, is more commonly associated with Juvéderm. In those with thin, translucent skin, the blueness is distractingly obvious. Nowadays I find myself removing more misplaced Juvéderm from under the eyes than insertion of Restylane.

Both products are also manufactured in a more robust version that is intended for deeper placement into the soft tissues with a potential for greater duration. Perlane, at the same concentration (20 mg/mL), is a version of Restylane with larger particle size, and Juvéderm Ultraplus, at the same concentration as Juvéderm, has greater viscosity.[4] However, I remain unconvinced that a clinically recognizable difference is appreciable between the more robust version and its less expensive version by the patient or me. More recently, I have been limiting my use to the Restylane or Juvéderm Ultra versions. However, I eagerly anticipate the arrival of the highly regarded large-particle Voluma and Restylane SubQ for facial shaping. In addition, Belotero (Merz Aesthetics, San Mateo, CA, USA), a smooth-consistency monophasic HA, seems likely to gain FDA approval soon, and is reported to provide correction without risk for a Tyndall effect because of its trademark cohesive polydensified matrix properties. This product may prove to be superior for treating the tear trough.

Calcium hydroxyapatite fillers

Radiesse (Merz Aesthetics, Inc, San Mateo, CA, USA), a biostimulating filler approved by the FDA in 2006, comprises calcium hydroxyapatite (CaHA) microspheres (30%) surrounded by a carboxy methylcellulose resorbable aqueous gel carrier (70%), leaving behind a matrix scaffolding of CaHA beads and setting up a potential framework for neocollagen deposition. Although I do not find the collagen inducting property to be clinically significant, I find CaHA to be a very reliable and safe product. Radiesse's high G′, indicating the product's firmness and ability to project tissues, is a major advantage for correcting deeper wrinkles and folds.[5] I find it particularly helpful for treating those with thicker skin and those who desire highlighting or emphasis of bony prominences such as malar, chin, and jawline areas. Its insignificant hydrophilic properties mean "what you see is what you get" after placing it, and any further augmentation is negligible. Therefore, it is important to realize that if not placed thinly or diffusely, it can result in hard streaks and nodules. I prefer to premix 0.3 mL of 1% lidocaine with epinephrine into the product just before treatment. This FDA-approved process not only makes the product more malleable but also reduces discomfort during placement.

In economic terms, most of the fillers are priced competitively; however, Radiesse contains 1.5 mL of product per syringe, compared with 0.8 mL and 1.0 mL for Juvéderm and Restylane, respectively. Although variations in retail pricing to the patient exist across the country, for most practices, Radiesse with the additional product per syringe may be a more economical option. It goes further for the dollar and this may be a deciding factor for some patients. Radiesse is not immediately reversible, whereas the effects from misplaced or excess HA can be reversed within 12 to 24 hours following an injection of hyaluronidase (Vitrase; ISTA Pharmaceuticals, Irvine, CA, USA). This factor may be an influence on the inexperienced filler patient or doctor.

Poly-L-lactic acid

Poly-L-lactic acid (Sculptra; Sanofi Aventis, Bridgewater, NJ, USA) received FDA approval for cosmetic use in 2009. It is a product that relies on its controlled foreign-body biostimulatory properties, and is preferred by many physicians and patients for its subtle and progressive augmentation. However, too robust of a response can be problematic, resulting in nodules and, rarely, granulomas.[6] I target this product for a small niche of patients requesting global facial volumization. I often prefer fat in such situations, but in thin individuals lacking adequate fat stores for harvesting or in human immunodeficiency virus patients with lipodystrophy, I find Sculptra to be the best and most appropriate filler. Although its augmenting benefits are slowly realized, they can be very impressive; but as the results are not immediate, patients' expectations have to be well managed. In an era of immediate gratification, the necessity to reconstitute with water days in advance and having to do a series of treatments to recognize the benefits make this product less user-friendly than other off-the-shelf fillers.

Silicone and polymethylmethacrylate

Other fillers that I use less often include the permanent silicone (Silikon 1000 purified polydimethylsiloxane; Alcon Laboratories, Fort Worth, TX, USA) and polymethylmethacrylate (PMMA) (Artefill; Suneva, San Diego, CA, USA). I find the hardness properties of these products very advantageous for filling in the fine rhytids of the upper lip, scars, and deep etched-in dermal rhytids. However, silicone's long-term questionable side effects prevent me from selecting it in younger patients, the lip bodies, or those with thicker skin. Artefill comprises PMMA beads surrounded by a bovine collagen, and in 2006 became the only permanent FDA-approved filler product in the United States. However, it has had difficulty gaining popularity. Its properties are impressive, as is its 5-year safety data.[7] I use this product for deeper etched-in wrinkles of the face in those insistent on a permanent solution.

ELLIS

At present, there is no universally accepted classification system for injectable fillers but they can be categorized into the following parameters: type of filler, method of action, and duration of action. Fillers can be either biodegradable or nonbiodegradable. The source of the filler may be natural/animal, synthetic, or natural synthetic. Method of action can be based on replacement of volume or stimulator of fibroplasia and collagen, or both. The duration of action may be temporary, semipermanent, or permanent. Patients are more interested in their duration of the filler in the specific areas they wish to be augmented.

Indications can be viewed as filler-based and patient-based depending on the characteristics of each filler and where the filler is to be injected. For instance, in the tear troughs, I like to use a minimal amount of filler that is not stiff. HA-based fillers work well in this area. Several pitfalls, however, may occur in this area:

1. Too superficial an injection can result in a bluish hue under thin skin, known as the Tyndall effect.
2. Too much volume can result in lumpiness and exacerbation of bags under the eyes, especially when the patient is smiling.

I have used Juvéderm Refine, Juvéderm Ultra Plus with Lidocaine, and Juvéderm Ultra with Lidocaine for this area. Juvéderm Voluma (20 mg/mL total HA concentration) is too viscous and thick to inject in the tear trough, periorbital areas, or lips, but is an ideal product for the cheek and chin. Juvéderm Voluma has been approved for use in Canada but is still under clinical investigation in the United States. As one of the initial clinical investigators of this product in Canada, we have seen tremendous results in patients requiring volume replacement for facial rejuvenation. I find the product easy to inject (although it is noticeably firmer and requires more force to inject than traditional high molecular weight [MW] HAs), to sculpt, and to mold. It is well tolerated by patientsl as evidenced by their satisfaction with the product, likelihood of returning for additional treatment, and their willingness to recommend the product to others. However, I have injected into the lips and the patients have not felt it to be too stiff or firm. In previous years, Gore-Tex is been used to insert the lips for a permanent filler, and Gore-Tex is much firmer than Voluma. Patients enjoy the length of time Voluma lasts.

The added benefit of using an HA-based filler is that it can be dissolved out with hyaluronidase if the patient is unhappy with the product. In areas where inadvertent skin necrosis is a concern, hyaluronidase is essential in one's armamentarium to treat such a disastrous complication.

Defects to be corrected by fillers as a first choice include the NLF, marionette and oral commissural lines, labiomental crease, mid-cheeks/zygoma, chin, lips, philtrum, ear lobe, tear trough, infrabrow, temporal depressions, and hands. In young Asian patients, we have used fillers to augment the dorsum of the nose, project the nasal tip, and occasionally have placed filler in the nasal spine to allow increased tip rotation. Fillers can also be used for dynamic wrinkles of the upper face and vertical wrinkles of the white lip, but are less effective that other rejuvenation techniques available such as Botox or laser resurfacing. Sites where fillers are not indicated would include nonextensible scars, neck and necklines, and sites of previously implanted permanent or unknown fillers. One exception to this would be our clinical experience of HA fillers in patients with previously implanted Bio-Alcamid (Polymekon, Brindisi, Italy), a nonabsorbable hydropolymer used as injectable permanent filler for cosmetic treatment and soft-tissue reconstructive defects.

MORAN

With our enhanced understanding of the role of fillers in panfacial rejuvenation, the indication for fillers has expanded. Even without any significant changes in technology of the fillers themselves, we have a greater appreciation of their varied applications.

I use lighter, less viscous HA products near the surface of the skin and in tear troughs. I use heavier, more viscous products in the deeper subcutaneous layers and to augment fat and bony deficiencies in the face. I often layer them when appropriate.

In your opinion, what are the durations of the various fillers?

DAYAN

Duration of the products varies not only between the individual filler types, but also can be highly variable amongst its own brand. The HAs absorb water, gaining additional correction after being injected. HAs are reversible, metabolized via enzymatic degradation and reaction with a reactive oxygen species,[3] and have FDA approval for 12 months on initial treatment with Juvéderm and 18 months with retreatment for Restylane. However, many experienced practitioners acknowledge incidences of correction that have extended well beyond 1 year. In fact, I have many patients in whom fullness and/or visible product is still evident at 3 years or longer. By contrast, I have others in whom it is completely resorbed within 3 months.

The reason some patients retain fillers and others rapidly metabolize it remains elusive. However, I believe a few factors beyond the individual patient's metabolism contribute to the duration of the product. If placed into a confined nonmobile space, the product seems to last longer. I have many patients in whom I have placed a small quantity, less than 0.2 mL, into the tight space between the thick superficial musculoaponeurotic system and thin periosteum above the bony nasal dorsum, and the correction has persisted beyond 2 years. A 2007 report from the University of Michigan showed that HA can stimulate collagen production,[8] perhaps contributing to its extended correction. In addition, I have seen many patients with worm-like lumps and bumps in the immobile NLF dermis from product placed years prior. I am certain the product is in the dermis because without any bleeding, it is easily expressed after puncturing the skin with an 18-gauge needle. It is interesting that the HA filler looks exactly like it did before being injected.

I also believe that, if placed in large quantities or if an early retreatment is given, the product seems to last longer. In 2010, we published data showing persistence of correction at 36 months with retreatment in the NLF.[9] Although shown not to experience the fibrous ingrowth like the permanent hydrogels,[10] it seems the HAs, with their very thin fibrous capsule, can develop a homeostatic and synergistic relationship with the surrounding tissue exchanging metabolites. Also, perhaps in greater quantities or concentration, the enlarged surface area results in inefficient metabolism of the product.[3] I do not recognize any differences in persistence between Juvéderm and Restylane and routinely tell patients they can expect between 6 months to a year from the product, with it lasting longer in some people and shorter in others.

CaHA is metabolized by enzymatic breakdown with absorption of microspheres evident at 9 months.[11] I find CaHA lasts predictably and routinely from 9 to 12 months, regardless of the patient. However, I did have one patient who was taking ibandronate (Boniva; Roche Therapeutics Inc, Nutley, NJ, USA) and she felt that it dissipated quicker. However, I cannot confirm this nor have I seen any scientific validation.

Poly-L-lactic acid is likely degraded by hydrolysis and extracellular enzymes, and subsequently broken down by macrophages.[11] In my experience, it can be expected to last from 12 to 18 months following a series of 3 treatments. It is difficult, however, to gauge its persistence because the correction is so gradual and diffuse.

Artefill does provide for appreciable permanent results. However, in the NLF, where I have the most experience with the product, it seems necessary to gain complete correction first with multiple syringes, 2.0 to 3.0 mL.

ELLIS

Temporary fillers are usually resorbed by the body in about 6 months to 1 year. Semipermanent fillers may last 1 to 2 years. Permanent fillers are basically nonresorbable.

Temporary fillers include:

1. Bovine-derived collagen (Zyderm, Zyplast)
2. Allogenic collagen (Cosmoderm, Cosmoplast, Cymetra, Fascian)
3. Synthetic HA materials (Juvéderm Refine/Ultra/ Ultra Plus, Restylane and Perlane, Teosyal, Esthelis, Isogel, Belotero).

Semipermanent fillers are often alloplastic in nature with the exception of Juvéderm Voluma. These fillers include:

  Radiesse: an aqueous-based gel carrier with spherical particles of synthetic CaHA

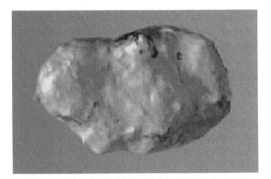

Fig. 2. Juvéderm Voluma. Juvéderm Voluma is a smooth but highly cohesive and viscous gel. (*Courtesy of* Allergan Canada, Inc.)

Sculptra: a biodegradable poly-ʟ-lactic acid polymer

BeautiCal: known as Outline in Europe, an absorbable polyacrylamide gel.

Juvéderm Voluma is unique in that it confers all the advantages of HA-based fillers while providing greater longevity. Juvéderm Voluma is a smooth but highly cohesive and viscous gel that uses a combination of high-MW and low-MW HA polymer chains (**Fig. 2**). The addition of these low-MW chains improves the effectiveness of cross-linking, resulting in a product that is both cohesive and viscous (**Fig. 3**). In vitro, this translates to a product that is able to retain its structure and resists migration.

At present, Artefill is the only FDA-approved permanent injectable filler for facial soft tissues. Artefill received FDA approval in only 2006 although its predecessors, Arteplast and Artecoll, have been available for over a decade outside the United States. This product consists of PMMA microspheres suspended in 3.5% bovine collagen solution and 0.3% lidocaine.

Liquid silicone was the first highly popularized permanent injectable filler. It is a colorless and odorless product composed of long chains of polymerized dimethylsiloxane. It was well accepted because of its natural feel and ease of injection. It was also well tolerated in small volumes. However, widespread use led to recognition of a fibrotic reaction followed by low-grade inflammation and subsequent capsule formation. Publicized tragedies of organ failure and death from granulomatous hepatitis, pulmonary embolism, and silicone pneumonitis led to the withdrawal of silicone by the FDA in 1991. At present, silicone oil is approved by the FDA only for ophthalmic use.

Polyalkylimide hydrogels have also been marketed as permanent fillers, the most popular being Bio-Alcamid. Bio-Alcamid is a nonabsorbable hydropolymer composed of 96% apyrogenic water and 4% polyalkylimide. It is currently not FDA approved, but has been available in Europe since 2001 and Health Canada approved since 2006. Two other permanent hydrogel fillers used for cosmetic facial contouring include Aquamid from Denmark and Argiform from Russia. Both are polyacrylamide polymers of different consistencies.

One must also consider that the mobility of the area in which filler is injected can have significant impact on its duration; this pertains especially to temporary fillers. In mobile areas, such as the NLF and lips, HA fillers will last up to 6 months before reinjection is needed, whereas in immobile

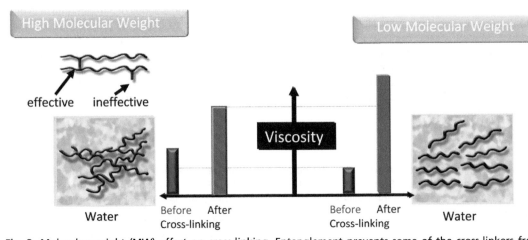

Fig. 3. Molecular weight (MW) effect on cross-linking. Entanglement prevents some of the cross-linkers from binding 2 chains together ("ineffective" cross-linking). Greater amount of effective cross-linking in the low-MW solution results in more viscous gel, even though it started out less viscous than high-MW hyaluronic acid. (*Courtesy of* Allergan Canada, Inc.)

areas such as the cheeks, the prejowl sulcus, earlobes, temples, and angle of jaw, longevity of the product approaches 12 months. According to both clinician and patient assessment, Juvéderm Voluma in the cheek area is reported to last for up to 18 months after treatment before reinjection is needed.

MORAN

It depends on the location and the amount of correction performed at the time of treatment. It also depends on whether there is previous treatment to the area. Perhaps smoking plays a role. I find, also, that it seems to holds less well in patients who are already deficient in facial fat. I would guesstimate that Restylane holds 6 to 12 months, Perlane 9 to 18 months, and Juvéderm 9 to 18 months. I don't yet have any experience with Radiesse or Sculptra. I am not certain how much permanent correction I saw when I was using Artefill. Certainly there was some, but I felt like I saw a diminution over time.

Is there still a role for the use of collagen injections?

DAYAN

Collagen (Zyderm; Inamed, Santa Barbara, CA, USA) was the first FDA-approved bovine filler in 1981 for cosmetic use and enjoyed 20 years of a filler monopoly. Much was learned about the risks and benefits of cosmetic correction with the collagens. Its properties were well liked for filling in fine wrinkles and folds, and it worked well when placed into the deep dermis. However, the need to postpone an initial treatment because of skin testing and its limited persistence contributed to its demise. Skin testing was not necessary for the human-based collagens (Dermalogen and Cosmoderm/Cosmoplast), but similar to the bovine collagen, duration was limited to 12 weeks. The collagens were quickly crowded out when Restylane became the first FDA-approved HA for cosmetic use in December 2003. The greater than 1000% rapid increase in HA use from 116,000 injections in 2003 to 1.3 million injections in 2010[1] attests to its increased popularity and greater acceptance among physicians and patients. Collagen, however, retained a limited role because many practitioners still favored Cosmoderm for the vermilion border until it was discontinued in late 2010.

There was a brief resurgence in collagen popularity with the June 2008 FDA approval for the porcine-derived collagen product Evolence (Colbar LifeSciences/Johnson & Johnson, New Brunswick, NJ, USA). Skin testing was unnecessary and a 12-month cosmetically appealing correction of an NLF could be expected. Unfortunately, the product did not achieve its business objectives and was discontinued in 2009. In my practice, there is no role currently for collagen products. I can achieve fine-detail correction of superficial rhytids with Restylane or silicone, and the collagens are not indicated for deeper facial shaping.

ELLIS

Although collagen injections have an effective and safe 30-year history of clinical use, I do not currently use any collagen injections. I believe that HA products have been shown in numerous studies to be more durable and safer.

Unfortunately, there is still much debate over which product is the ideal filler, although we can all agree that the perfect filler should be:

1. Safe, first and foremost
2. Effective
3. Painless
4. Nonanimal
5. Long lasting
6. Natural
7. Comfortable to inject
8. Cost effective.

Capital demand from both physicians and patients will drive market forces to develop prospective fillers to meet these purposes. Over time the fillers with poor safety profiles, suboptimal results, and significant complications will cease to exist.

MORAN

There is a role for collagen and I am very disappointed that it no longer exists. I have patients who would only use collagen. It is great for fine superficial lines. I hope they come back to the market.

What complications concern you and what do you do in your practice to attempt to avoid or minimize these?

DAYAN

The 2 most concerning complications following filler treatments are:

1. Vascular compromise
2. Hypersensitivity reactions

Impending necrosis

Although soft-tissue filler necrosis is rare, with HA and collagen incidences estimated at 0.001%,[12,13] it poses a serious complication and may be more common in vascular watershed areas such as the NLF or the glabella. Vascular compromising complications associated with soft-tissue fillers can be categorized by time of onset, and it has been my experience that manifestation of impending necrosis either occurs immediately, or early (within 24–48 hours of injection), or is delayed. Although each presentation requires a slightly different treatment regimen, I have had success in preventing significant scarring or sequelae. All physicians should be aware of a treatment protocol.

Immediate intravascular injection of product and occlusion is likely a causation of necrosis, which is apparent by an immediate blanching along a recognizable vascular pattern. Aspirating before injecting may be helpful to indentifying intravascular cannulization, but it is technically difficult to achieve sufficient aspiration with the current FDA-approved cosmetic soft-tissue filler products. In my practice, I perform a slower injection (<0.3 mL/min), keep the needle in motion, and avoid injection in the immediate vicinity of large facial vessels. Furthermore, to minimize the risk for occlusion, I premix our product with 0.3 mL of lidocaine before injection to decrease its viscosity. However, the likely causes of most the impending necrosis reported is the result of pressure necrosis secondary to local edema or the hydrophilic properties of the product occluding vessels, explaining the delayed onset.

I have instituted a modified version of a previous published protocol[14] to treat all versions of impending necrosis subsequent to soft-tissue filler injection, with efficacious results (**Table 1**). Apparent blanching followed by a dusky or purple discoloration of the injection area is an indicator of vascular compromise, and the injection should be immediately discontinued.[15] Ten to 30 units of hyaluronidase (Vitrase; ISTA Pharmaceuticals, Irvine, CA, USA) diluted 1:1 with saline per 2 × 2-cm area should be injected into the area of impending necrosis, regardless of type of filler injected. With hyaluronidase, hypersensitivity reaction can occur and skin testing should be performed before injection.[15–17] Hyaluronidase has edema-reducing benefits, and has been efficacious in mediating rejection-induced edema[18] and necrosis associated with myocardial infarction.[19,20] It is probable that the increased inflammatory response causes an increase in hyaluronan due to proinflammatory cytokines and growth factors, which is then

Table 1
Recognition and management of impending necrosis

Presentation	Immediate or early blanching followed by a dusky or purple discoloration of the area
Treatment	Discontinue injection Perform hyaluronidase skin testing Inject 10–30 U of hyaluronidase per 2 × 2-cm area Massage 0.5 inch of 2% nitroglycerin paste into the area. Apply warm compresses Begin 325 mg aspirin and an antacid regimen Apply topical oxygen cosmeceutical therapy twice a day
Further management	Follow patient daily for further signs of occlusion/necrosis Continue hyaluronidase and 2% nitroglycerin paste daily as needed Continue aspirin, antacid, and topical oxygen therapy until wound has healed If edema progresses, place on Medrol Dose pack Consider hyperbaric oxygen for progressing necrosis resistant to the above treatment options

mitigated by the hyaluronidase.[21–25] Its edema-reducing benefits and theoretical reduction in occluding vessel pressure is why I believe it is efficacious in treating impending necrosis secondary to all products, not just HA.

In addition, 2% nitroglycerin paste (Nitro-BID; E. Fougera & Co., Melville, NY, USA) is applied to the affected area with the amount dependent on size and area of impending necrosis. The nitroglycerin paste is applied daily to the affected area so long as the capillary refill rate is less than 2 seconds. Warm compresses are applied and the area is massaged to increase vasodilation. An immediate vasodilatory effect with improvement in the skin color is often realized. Care is taken to use a small amount of 2% nitroglycerin paste (approximately 0.5 inch), as excess can lead to unwanted systemic effects.

An aspirin regimen of 325 mg daily is started to prevent further clot formation, and an antacid is used to reduce the risk for aspirin-associated gastritis. Topical oxygen cosmeceutical therapy (Dermacyte Oxygen Concentrate; Oxygen Biotherapeutics, Inc, Durham, NC, USA) is applied to the affected area twice daily. Topical oxygen therapies have demonstrated an enhanced rate of epithelialization of excisional wounds and second-degree burns.[26] Depending on the severity of the condition, hyperbaric oxygen may also be recommended as a treatment option for impending necrosis.[12,27] However, the risks, benefits, and inconveniences associated with the treatment may pose significant barriers to some, and the procedure is recommended in instances of severe necrosis or delayed presentations in which the tissue is not healing well.[15]

Patients are followed daily for further signs of occlusion or necrosis. Nitroglycerin paste massages can be stopped if improvement is noted; however, they anecdotally seem to accelerate the reticulated vascular congestion resolution. Topical oxygen therapy and aspirin are continued until the wound is satisfactorily healed. If there is no improvement or progression of necrosis occurs, the regimen should be repeated daily. If edema is slow to resolve, methylprednisolone (Medrol Dosepak; Pfizer, New York, NY, USA) is added. Hyperbaric oxygen should be considered the aforementioned measures are still not adequate.

Hypersensitivity or infectious reactions

Before 1999, the reported rate of hypersensitivity reactions following HA was 0.07%.[12,28–32] Following the introduction of a more highly purified product containing lower amounts of protein, the incidence of hypersensitivity reactions decreased to 0.02%.[29] Other commonly used fillers such as CaHA and poly-L-lactic acid have also been associated with hypersensitivity reactions.[14]

Hypersensitivity reactions following the use of non-permanent filler treatments are poorly understood, yet frequently reported in the literature. The classic Type IV, T-cell mediated delayed hypersensitivity reaction occurs following exposure to a foreign antigen and involves the upregulation of the mediators of inflammation and recruitment of macrophages and leukocytes. A classic Type I hypersensitivity response should include antibody formation and predispose the patient to an equal or greater immunologic response following a second exposure to the sensitizing material. Reports supporting either mechanism are sparse, and the follow-up evaluations to confirm the occurrence of immune-related events are usually negative. The titles of several reports suggest immediate or delayed immune-mediated reactions following the use of HA fillers despite a paucity of documented evidence.[33] These reported hypersensitivity reactions might be secondary to an infectious process.[34]

Bacteria are incredibly tenacious and are probably the most adaptive organism known. Their ability to continuously adapt and evolve as they become increasingly resistant to growing numbers of antibiotics is well known.[35] Bacteria may do this by forming a biofilm, reducing their metabolism, cell-to-cell signaling, and secreting a protective extracellular HA and polymorphic glycocalyx matrix, which prevents white blood cell penetration.[36–38] The nature of the protective matrix may explain the reason why the use of hyaluronidase has been successful for the treatment of reactions caused by non-HA dermal fillers.

Biofilms can present as sterile abscess or chronic indolent inflammation and infections.[39] There have been multiple confirmed reports of biofilm reactions in FDA-unapproved permanent dermal fillers, whereas confirmed reactions have yet to be reported in approved nonpermanent fillers currently in use in the United States today.

However, the symptoms and clinical course of most reported hypersensitivity and granulomatous reactions following filler treatments appear to be inconsistent with a hypersensitivity reaction and are more consistent with an infectious etiology. It has been shown that hydrogel fillers contaminated with bacteria can cause a foreign-body response, mimicking an allergic reaction.[34,40] Oral and/or intralesional steroids and nonsteroidal anti-inflammatory drugs (NSAIDs) are routinely used as first-line agents to treat hyperinflammatory conditions such as Type I and Type IV hypersensitivity reactions; however, the treatment of inflammation secondary to an infectious biofilm with steroids and NSAIDs has been associated with a worse outcome and prolongation of the infectious biofilm. The steroids and NSAIDs mask the contamination by providing a brief reduction in inflammation; however, the biofilm continues to thrive and encapsulate itself from the surrounding host tissues.[41] It thereby increases its resistance and remains ready to resurface after steroids and NSAIDs are discontinued.

Successful treatments of early infectious complications from biofilm reactions have included high-dose administration of a prolonged course of broad-spectrum antibiotics such as fluoroquinolone (ciprofloxacin, levofloxacin) or macrolide (azithromycin, clarithromycin) antibiotics.[37] Sterile technique together with prophylactic measures before or immediately following treatment with permanent fillers can reduce the risk for infectious complication.[42]

It is my impression that hypersensitivity reactions are more likely of infectious than immunologic etiology. Therefore, I have instituted specific measures to be avoided and protocols to treat hypersensitivity/infectious reactions (**Table 2**).

As the use of fillers becomes increasingly more common and the skill level of those injecting is so varied, adverse events can be expected to increase as well. Avoiding complications is always the best measure, and with appropriate training and injection techniques many complications can be avoided. However, adverse events can occur in the best of hands, and early detection is imperative. If a consensus can be agreed on how to treat adverse events effectively, devastating complications can be avoided.

ELLIS

The most common complications I have seen are:

1. Bruising
2. Reactivation of herpes simplex around the mouth
3. Skin necrosis around the nasal tip
4. Long-term infections with Bio-Alcamid

To minimize bruising, I use a quiet needle technique whereby the tip of the needle is not moved

Table 2
Preventing and treating hypersensitivity/infections reactions

Before treatment	Cleanse the face thoroughly of all makeup before injection Use benzalkonium chloride wash or betadine swab to prepare the face just before the treatment Use as few injection sites as possible Avoid bolus injections Avoid injecting into previously placed fillers or through infected tissue Avoid injecting through oral or nasal mucosa Consider prophylactic antibiotics before a dental procedure or if a facial infection occurs within 2 weeks of a filler treatment
If a red indurated area appears any time after the treatment, regardless of duration	Inject hyaluronidase (Vitrase; ISTA Pharmaceuticals, Irvine, CA, USA) regardless of filler used 10–30 units mixed 1:1 with saline Start antibiotics Ciprofloxacin 500 mg every day (Cipro; Bayer HealthCare Pharmaceuticals, Inc. Wayne, NJ, USA) and clarithromycin 500 mg twice a day (Biaxin; Abbott Laboratories, Abbott Park, IL, USA) Avoid all forms of steroids or nonsteroidal anti-inflammatories
If long-term indurated area and/or steroids have already been used	Inject fluorouracil 15–40 mg (APP Pharmaceuticals, LLC, Schaumburg, IL, USA) Repeat every 4 weeks
If induration remains persistent despite 5-fluorouracil treatment	Consider laser lysis Consider incision and washing out cavity with antibiotics Surgical excision as last resort

very much. I have patients discontinue aspirin, vitamin E, and ginkgo 2 weeks before injections. Using the smallest-gauge needle that will accommodate injection flow of the product is also helpful. Furthermore, I often use an anterograde injection technique, which allows me to introduce small amounts of product ahead of the needle as to bluntly shift blood vessels away from the bevel. Some of my patients take homeopathic medications such as Arnica pellets and topical gel to prevent and hasten resolution of bruising.

With lip injections and those who have a history of herpes simplex, I often prescribe Valtrex or a comparable antiviral to start the day before injection, and continue for 5 days afterward. I have not found it necessary to pretreat when correcting marionette or oral commissural lines.

Injections around the alar groove of the nose have been known to cause skin necrosis (Fig. 4); this has happened to me and I stopped further injection. It is my feeling that the speed of injection

in this area should be very gentle, and a retrograde technique is used to augment this area. With post-rhinoplasty tip asymmetry being corrected with HAs, I think it is important to do a very slow injection, watching the skin for blanching and exquisite sharp pain. If this should occur, nitro-paste applied topically can be very effective in minimizing permanent scarring.

To date I have treated 21 patients with late Bio-Alcamid infections. In working with the Infectious Disease Department at our tertiary medical center, we have identified several patients treated with Bio-Alcamid in the greater Toronto area presenting with these infections as late as 3 to 4 years out. Although not identifiable in every case, we have anecdotally identified dental procedures as a common triggering event in one-third of these cases. I recommend antibiotic prophylaxis to all our personal patients (Keflex 1000 mg 1 hour before a dental procedure, even teeth cleaning) for the rest of their life.

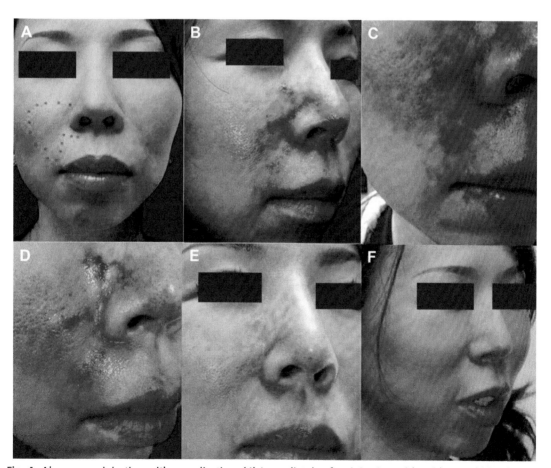

Fig. 4. Alar groove injection with complication. (*A*) Immediately after injection with evidence of blanching of overlying skin (*outline in red dots*). Injection was stopped immediately. (*B*) Twenty-four hours postinjection. (*C*) Forty-eight hours postinjection. (*D*) Five days postinjection. (*E*) Nine days postinjection. (*F*) Two weeks postinjection, with no permanent sequelae.

MORAN

Certainly bruising is a pesky side effect. We try to remind patients not to take any nonsteroidals, fish oil, flax seed oil, or vitamin E for 2 weeks prior. We also recommend that patients minimize their alcohol intake for a few days prior. All of these apply afterward as well. We do give them Arnica Montana if bruising seems likely. Most importantly, we counsel them not to schedule their treatment right before important personal or professional commitments so as not to put them in an awkward position.

We do not let patients use makeup for the evening after their treatment in order to avoid infection. In terms of any more serious side effects, we try to avoid overinjecting and have hyaluronidase handy in case the treatment needs to be reversed.

What type of anesthesia do you use, when, and why?

DAYAN

The choice of anesthesia when treating patients with fillers varies based on the individual patient, the product used, and the area being treated. Since early 2010, both Restylane and Juvéderm have been manufactured with 0.3% dry preservative-free lidocaine, which has significantly reduced discomfort during and immediately following the injection.[43] However, in my practice I premix filler products with 1% lidocaine regardless. Consequently, the newer fillers have not had a significant impact on my treatment protocols. I believe that by premixing with lidocaine, the filler viscosity is significantly reduced, further contributing to its anesthetic effectiveness. In addition, I have converted to using almost exclusively blunt-tip cannulas (SoftFil; AlphaMedix, Petah Tikva, Israel), which cause much less discomfort than traditional needles. When treating the cheeks and tear trough, there is very little discomfort and I find anesthetic unnecessary.

For those who are highly pain averse when treating the lower one-third of the face, especially the lips, I anesthetize with a regional nerve block. My continuously evolving technique starts by placing a topical cotton tip swabbed 2% benzocaine paste (Hurricane Beutlich Pharmaceuticals, Waukegan, IL, USA) along the oral buccal mucosal, followed 5 minutes later with 4 intraoral injections of isocaine (Mepivicaine HCl 3%; Henry Schein, Melville, NY, USA), 2 superior and 2 inferior, anesthetizing the labial branches of the inferior orbital nerve and the mental nerves. Isocaine, with its basic pH and short-acting duration (approximately 30 minutes), is better tolerated than the acidic and prolonged numbing lidocaine.

A valuable pearl is to place a vibrating nerve distracter cutaneously near and above the injection point during injection of isocaine, which works incredibly well at confusing sensory recognition of the injection. Patients often are unaware where they have been injected. Most recently, I have become increasingly satisfied with anesthetic effects achieved with topical 30% lidocaine cream (SCP, Sherman Oaks, CA, USA). Although the topical has to remain in place for 20 to 30 minutes before adequate anesthesia is realized, it is an appropriate alternative for those who are resistant to injection nerve blocks. However, on the NLF I have found topical anesthetics to be of modest benefit. For the lips, I have been very impressed with the level of anesthesia achieved by placing topical cream into a specially designed mouth guard, concentrating the product over the highly absorbent labial mucosa.

ELLIS

I do not normally use any other local anesthetic other than what is in the product (ie, Juvéderm Ultra Plus with lidocaine). After entry of the skin with the needle bevel, typically I will deposit a small droplet of product and wait 3 seconds. Often this short period of time is sufficient to dull the pain as I proceed with anterograde injection technique. I also make it a point to stagger my injection sites so that I enter through an area that has already been injected, to take advantage of the local anesthetic effect. For instance, I will inject starting at the inferior aspect of the nasolabial fold and work up superiorly.

We find that ice packs before and after injection are helpful in pain relief. Distraction techniques, such as massage, verbal coaching, and slow breathing, are also interventions that are effective, inexpensive, and easy to implement.

If patients are having Voluma (not yet commercially available with local anesthetic) injected into their lips, I do an intramuscular lip block to alleviate the pain of injection while preserving the landmarks of the lip.

Although not available in Canada any more, the injection of Bio-Alcamid requires a 14- to 18-gauge needle and, therefore, local anesthetic is needed only where the needle penetrates the skin. The entry site should be away from the area to be augmented, so as to minimize volume distortion.

MORAN

For most fillers we apply a lidocaine 23%/tetracaine 7% gel that is formulated by a local pharmacy. Patients generally sit with it on their face for 30 minutes in the office before treatment. If we are injecting their lips, we perform nerve blocks of V2 and V3 nerve as well as a sublabial block.

Analysis: Over the past 5 years, how have you modified your techniques or approach or what is the most important thing you have learned/observed in working with injectables and fillers?

DAYAN

Since I began teaching an undergraduate course at DePaul University on "The Science of Beauty and its Impact on Culture," my philosophy, evaluation, and cosmetic treatment techniques have changed significantly. Understanding that beauty works as a subliminal form of evolutionary communication used to depict our health and vitality is critical to successful treatment of patients.

Primitive neural pathways in the amygdala and posterior cingulate cortex process facial characteristics[44] and determine an emotional response that allows humans to make accurate judgments[44–46] within 39 to 100 milliseconds.[45,46] Previously, I have reported that those who undergo facial plastic surgery, botulinum neuromodulators, and hyaluronic fillers project a more favorable first impression to unknowing observers.[47–49] However, it is important that the alteration and message of beauty remains subconsciously communicated. An obviously overdone cosmetic change actually has the opposite effect of its intent, clueing in the unknowing observer that a genetic weakness exists. As cosmetic physicians we may possess the skill, talent, and tools to improve one's physical appearance. However, it is equally important, if not more so, to know what makes someone attractive and why.

Symmetry
Throughout nature, symmetric individuals have faster growth rates, higher fecundity, and better survival rates than asymmetric individuals.[50] From an evolutionary perspective, the more symmetric a face is, the more likely is it disease free.[51] The closer the facial characteristic is to the midline, the more important symmetry is to influencing the level of attractiveness.[52]

The eyes
Humans are the only primates to have white sclera, which allows one to visualize another's pupils.[53] Enormous amounts of information are gained from visualizing someone's eyes. In a 2010 eye-tracking study, observers were asked to look and judge the appearance of photographed individuals. The facial feature most commonly looked at first was the eyes.[54]

The importance of the eyes in making one appear attractive is essential to subliminal beauty, and after symmetry, most of our efforts in facial rejuvenation should be directed toward highlighting and accentuating the eyes. In keeping with this strategy, botulinum neuromodulators can be effective tools to elevate the brows, opening the eyelid aperture, and allowing the eyes to appear larger, more inviting, and attractive. Fillers have an increasingly important role to mitigate lower eyelid contour defects, raising the cheek lid pedestal and rejuvenating the brows: in essence, framing the eyes.

Lower third of face
Emphasizing the cheeks and narrowing the jaw by masking or reducing the squaring jowls, shrinking the defining masseters, and deemphasizing the lower one-third of the face are techniques that fit within the subliminal strategy to make a female face more attractive. A narrow, smaller lower third is a sexually defining dimorphic physical trait. Females are considered more attractive if they have large eyes, small chins, and defined, but petite, jawlines.[55] However, perhaps because of ease of treatment, standardized scales, and FDA indications, our attention and needles have turned primarily toward the nasolabial fold as a region necessary to treat. However, this is the opposite of what makes a female face attractive and is rather indicative of the masculine trait of a larger chin and square mandible. An overfilled, simian perioral region is contrary to the evolutionary strategy of beauty, which is to deemphasize the lower third.

Lips

A smaller facial framework also works to highlight the lips, which serve an important evolutionary role for signaling female fertility and are generally fuller in times of heightened fecundity.[56] During ovulation a female's lips swell slightly, yet sufficiently enough for a male to recognize subconsciously. Therefore, a subtle plumping of the lip borders and vermilion mimics this heightened sense of fertility.

Homogeneous skin tone

Human eyes look for contrast, and to the human brain heterogeneous or mottled skin with dark spots, wrinkles, and brown patches is identifying of aging and disease. Therefore, in helping to deliver subliminal beauty, skin treated with laser, intense pulsed light, and various topical skin regimens promotes a pinkish homogeneous hue best mimicking health.

Advancements in treatment techniques

My recent adoption of blunt-tip cannulas (SoftFil) for injecting fillers is the essential tool to treating patients both technically and philosophically within subliminal strategies of beauty. I use them for correcting all areas of the face, from the lips to cheeks to the tear troughs. Not only am I able to shape the face by placing fillers deeper; patients look better immediately and the morbidity of a filler treatment is virtually eliminated (**Fig. 5** and Video demonstrating technique). The cannulas have resulted in a filler procedure evolving from a treatment aimed at filling in superficial rhytids and folds that is often associated with discomfort, ecchymoses, and edema to an instant subliminal beauty makeover with likely no downtime. The cannulas I prefer are 22-gauge and 70-mm length; they gently push underlying soft tissue out of the way as they are advanced through facial planes. Patient satisfaction is impressive, and the natural results are immediately remarkable. I have found that there is a learning curve to overcome along with essentials necessary to achieving consistent results. By thinning the product (Juvéderm, Restylane, or Radiesse) with the addition of 1% lidocaine (0.3 mL) to the filler, it becomes malleable and moldable. Moreover, after being deposited deeply, the filler can be massaged into place much like a sculptor achieves with clay.

Attractive features of the face, such as the eyes and lips, can be framed, highlighted, and emphasized. The soft and blunt nature of the cannula requires, at times, additional force to get through or around fibrous tissues. Although this is not painful to the patient, it can be unsettling to both the patient and doctor not accustomed to this sensation. However, I believe the overwhelming benefits of this newest advance in technique will change the way fillers are both marketed and sold, as well as the way in which physicians evaluate and treat cosmetic patients.

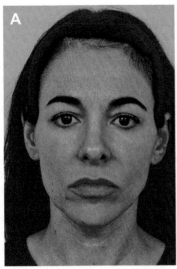
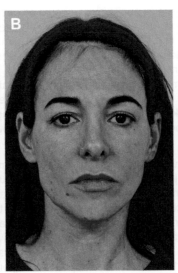
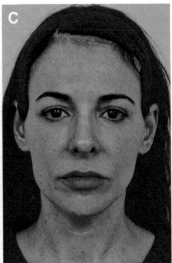

Fig. 5. Pretreatment (*A*), immediately after treatment (*B*), and 1 week following hyaluronic acid filler treatment (*C*) using blunt-tipped cannulas to the malar and temple areas.

ELLIS

I believe that it is important to counsel your patients that one session of injections will often not be sufficient to achieve optimal results. I ask that all my patients come back 2 weeks later for follow-up and possible touch-ups. This aspect is especially true when injecting tricky areas such as the lips because if the patient develops bruising and induration on one side, it is often near impossible to achieve perfect symmetry because it is difficult to estimate how much swelling is the result of the bruise versus filler.

Overlying skin necrosis is, fortunately, a very rare event. One needs to be skilled in identifying the early signs, as the more feared and detrimental complications can often be avoided. My one and only personal experience with this complication involved an injection rhinoplasty in a patient with a history of 3 previous rhinoplasties (**Fig. 6**). I would caution anyone attempting injectable filler in a previously operated field with a tenuous blood supply such as the nasal lobule. If one is to embark on such a challenge, the patient should be properly counseled on the risks and be educated in the signs and symptoms of impending skin necrosis so that he or she can seek medical treatment immediately.

In the past 5 years, I have also developed a system to remove certain permanent fillers. As previously discussed, in my practice I have encountered numerous Bio-Alcamid patients presenting with complaints of inflammation, hardening, migration, and even frank abscess formation. Conventional management of such complications typically involves oral antibiotic therapy followed by removal of the material. Unfortunately, we have seen patients treated with open incision and drainage as a last resort, leaving them with unsightly facial scars (**Fig. 7**). Because of the high volume of cosmetic patients referred to our practice for removal of previously implanted Bio-Alcamid and Artecoll, we have developed an in-office technique that facilitates safe and accurate removal of product with minimal risk of permanent scarring.

We pretreat all of our patients scheduled for Bio-Alcamid removal with at least 1 day of oral antibiotic therapy. Typically we start our patients on Keflex, 500 mg every day or clindamycin, 300 mg three times a day for penicillin-allergic patients. After local antiseptic cleaning with an alcohol swab, local anesthetic is infiltrated only in the area for needle entry, ideally located 5 to 7 mm inferior to the collection. A 14-gauge 1.5-inch needle on a 10-mL syringe is used to enter the skin and puncture the collagen capsule that surrounds the filler. The nondominant hand should be guiding the needle into the bulk of the product so that one succeeds in multiple piercings of the capsule. Of note, aspirating back on the syringe often removes little or no product. Unfortunately, this finding may come as a surprise to physicians who may stop any attempts at continued drainage at this point. In times of frank abscess formation, one is often successful in collecting purulent specimen in the syringe (**Fig. 8**).

Rarely do we send cultures unless pus is encountered, because often there is no identifiable bacterial growth. Antibiotics are only temporizing measures, because biofilms are believed to form on the capsule that encases the Bio-Alcamid filler. These biofilms are protected from the host's defenses and are adherent to the surface, which prevents the antibiotics from destroying the entire microorganism. As a result, bacteria are capable of surviving for extended periods when living within this proteinaceous biofilm, and serve as a source of infection when the opportunity arises.

Here is where technique may differ between Artecoll and Bio-Alcamid. Artecoll removal requires what I describe as an "apple-coring" motion through the lump, with needle and syringe on suction. Constant hand suction maintains pressure while the needle is within the bulk of the product. Typically one entry site is required, as the needle can be angled to remove product in multiple passes. This approach is particularly effective for nodules in the lip.

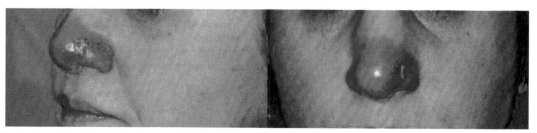

Fig. 6. Overlying left nasal tip necrosis in a patient with 3 previous rhinoplasties on day 3 postinjection.

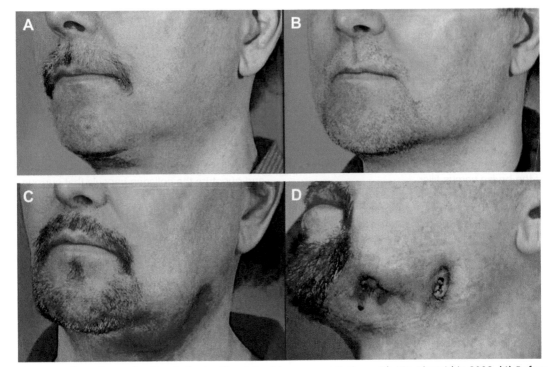

Fig. 7. Bio-Alcamid complication. Patient with angle of jaw augmentation with Bio-Alcamid in 2006. (*A*) Before filler augmentation. (*B*) After filler augmentation followed by infection 3 years later. (*C*) The patient sought medical care in an emergency room and underwent incision and drainage of "abscess." (*D*) Recalcitrant orocutaneous fistula 18 months after incision and drainage.

With Bio-Alcamid, the needle is removed and bimanual massage is used to manipulate the product out of the puncture site (**Fig. 9**). As it comes out, we have encountered either a granular gelatinous product tinged with a pink color or small fragmented clumps of filler intermixed with frank blood. We have found it very important to stress to patients that this technique will not remove all of the product, whether it is Artecoll or Bio-Alcamid. Most patients are treated with multiple

Fig. 8. Infected Bio-Alcamid syringe. Aspirated purulent material from facial abscess using a 10-mL syringe and large-bore 14-gauge 1.5-inch needle.

injections of Bio-Alcamid, so it is not uncommon to see one previously drained area reaccumulate with product from another tract, because there may be numerous tracts underneath the skin's surface connecting together pockets of Bio-Alcamid. Patients are counseled that they likely will need multiple treatments for further removal to even out resultant irregularities over time.

My patients continue oral antibiotic therapy for 5 days after the procedure, and I see them after 1 week for follow-up. The needle-entry site on average heals within 24 to 48 hours. To date, none of our patients treated with this approach have required intravenous antibiotics or open incision and drainage for recalcitrant infections. We have had no reports of remaining scar at the needle-entrance site, nor was this area problematic for any patients.

In working with injectable fillers for more than 25 years, I believe that as long as the pursuit for the perfect filler remains, the number of commercially available injectable soft-tissue fillers will continue to steadily increase. Only through extensive research and long-term clinical experience will we be able to answer this question. As the popularity of temporary fillers grow, more patients will seek out expert physicians for application of

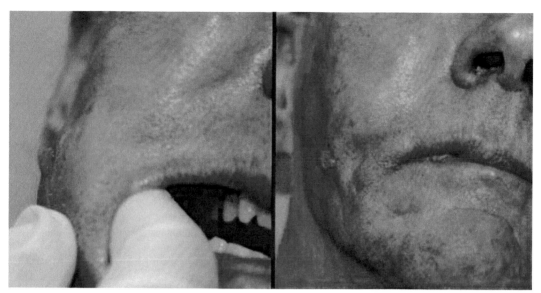

Fig. 9. Bio-Alcamid massage technique. After puncture of capsule, bimanual massage with constant pressure is needed to manipulate the product out of its subcutaneous tract.

longer-lasting soft-tissue enhancements. This challenge will continue to evolve, and I look forward to witnessing these new developments in hopes that I can one day offer my patients the ideal filler.

MORAN

Over the past 5 years working with injectables, I have gained an enhanced appreciation for how the face ages. Because of the versatility of fillers we have a greater ability to treat volume loss in places that we did not previously address, such as the temples, geniomandibular groove, tear trough, and orbitomalar junction. I am better able to address bony volume only in situations where I was able to use implants, which has been advantageous because it gives patients a chance to understand what kind of difference it would make before they commit to an implant. It is also addressing those patients who are averse to implants. I think that our experience with fillers has enabled us to notice volume changes in ways we never did previously, and that this has allowed us to enhance our surgical outcomes as well as reach an entirely broader group of patients that otherwise would not come to see us for surgery.

SUPPLEMENTARY DATA

Supplementary data related to this article can be found online at http://dx.doi.org/10.1016/j.fsc.2012.05.004.

REFERENCES: DAYAN

1. The American Society of Aesthetic Plastic Surgery. 2010 statistics from the American Society of Aesthetic Plastic Surgery, 2011. Available at: http://www.surgery.org/sites/default/files/Stats2010_1.pdf. Accessed April 26, 2011.

2. Carruthers J, Cohen SR, Joseph JH, et al. The science and art of dermal fillers for soft-tissue augmentation. J Drugs Dermatol 2009;8(4):335–50.

3. Kablik J, Monheit GD, Yu L, et al. Comparative physical properties of hyaluronic acid dermal fillers. Dermatol Surg 2009;35:302–12.

4. Gold M. Aesthetic update: what's new in fillers in 2010? J Clin Aesthet Dermatol 2010;3(8):36–45.

5. Sundaram H, Voigts B, Beer K, et al. Comparison of the rheological properties of viscosity and elasticity in two categories of soft tissue fillers: calcium hydroxylapatite and hyaluronic acid. Dermatol Surg 2010;36(Suppl 3):1859–65.

6. Hamilton DG, Gauthier N, Robertson BF. Late-onset, recurrent facial nodules associated with injection of poly-L-lactic acid. Dermatol Surg 2008;34(1):123–6.

7. Cohen SR, Berner CF, Busso M, et al. Five-year safety and efficacy of a novel polymethylmethacrylate aesthetic soft tissue filler for the correction of nasolabial folds. Dermatol Surg 2007;33(Suppl 2):S222–30.

8. Wang F, Garza LA, Kang S, et al. In vivo stimulation of de novo collagen production caused by crosslinked hyaluronic acid dermal filler injections in photodamaged human skin. Arch Dermatol 2007; 143(2):155–63.

9. Narins RS, Brandt FS, Dayan SH, et al. Persistence of nasolabial fold correction with a hyaluronic acid dermal filler with retreatment: results of an 18-month extension study. Dermatol Surg 2011; 37(5):644–50.

10. Fernandez-Cossio S, Castano-Oreja MT. Biocompatibility of two novel dermal fillers: histological evaluation of implants of a hyaluronic acid filler and a polyacrylamide filler. Plast Reconstr Surg 2006; 117(6):1789–96.

11. Lemperle G, Morhenn V, Charrier U. Human histology and persistence of various injectable filler substances for soft tissue augmentation. Aesthetic Plast Surg 2003;27(5):354–66 [discussion: 367].

12. Narins RS, Jewell M, Rubin M, et al. Clinical conference: management of rare events following dermal fillers—focal necrosis and angry red bumps. Dermatol Surg 2006;32(3):426–34.

13. Hanke CW, Higley HR, Jolivette DM, et al. Abscess formation and local necrosis after treatment with Zyderm or Zyplast collagen implant. J Am Acad Dermatol 1991;25(2 Pt 1):319–26.

14. Cohen JL. Understanding, avoiding, and managing dermal filler complications. Dermatol Surg 2008; 34(Suppl 1):S92–9.

15. Grunebaum LD, Bogdan Allemann I, Dayan S, et al. The risk of alar necrosis associated with dermal filler injection. Dermatol Surg 2009;35(Suppl 2):1635–40.

16. Hirsch RJ, Cohen JL, Carruthers JD. Successful management of an unusual presentation of impending necrosis following a hyaluronic acid injection embolus and a proposed algorithm for management with hyaluronidase. Dermatol Surg 2007; 33(3):357–60.

17. Brody HJ. Use of hyaluronidase in the treatment of granulomatous hyaluronic acid reactions or unwanted hyaluronic acid misplacement. Dermatol Surg 2005; 31(8 Pt 1):893–7.

18. Johnsson C, Hallgren R, Elvin A, et al. Hyaluronidase ameliorates rejection-induced edema. Transpl Int 1999;12(4):235–43.

19. Maroko PR, Hillis LD, Muller JE, et al. Favorable effects of hyaluronidase on electrocardiographic evidence of necrosis in patients with acute myocardial infarction. N Engl J Med 1977;296(16):898–903.

20. Maroko PR, Libby P, Bloor CM, et al. Reduction by hyaluronidase of myocardial necrosis following coronary artery occlusion. Circulation 1972;46(3): 430–7.

21. Engstrom-Laurent A, Feltelius N, Hallgren R, et al. Raised serum hyaluronate levels in scleroderma: an effect of growth factor induced activation of connective tissue cells? Ann Rheum Dis 1985;44(9):614–20.

22. Hamerman D, Wood DD. Interleukin 1 enhances synovial cell hyaluronate synthesis. Proc Soc Exp Biol Med 1984;177(1):205–10.

23. Heldin P, Laurent TC, Heldin CH. Effect of growth factors on hyaluronan synthesis in cultured human fibroblasts. Biochem J 1989;258(3):919–22.

24. Yaron M, Yaron I, Wiletzki C, et al. Interrelationship between stimulation of prostaglandin E and hyaluronate production by poly (I). poly (C) and interferon in synovial fibroblast culture. Arthritis Rheum 1978; 21(6):694–8.

25. Suzuki M, Asplund T, Yamashita H, et al. Stimulation of hyaluronan biosynthesis by platelet-derived growth factor-BB and transforming growth factor-beta 1 involves activation of protein kinase C. Biochem J 1995;307(Pt 3):817–21.

26. Davis SC, Cazzaniga AL, Ricotti C, et al. Topical oxygen emulsion: a novel wound therapy. Arch Dermatol 2007;143(10):1252–6.

27. Georgescu D, Jones Y, McCann JD, et al. Skin necrosis after calcium hydroxylapatite injection into the glabellar and nasolabial folds. Ophthal Plast Reconstr Surg 2009;25(6):498–9.

28. Sage RJ, Chaffins ML, Kouba DJ. Granulomatous foreign body reaction to hyaluronic acid: report of a case after melolabial fold augmentation and review of management. Dermatol Surg 2009; 35(Suppl 2):1696–700.

29. Friedman PM, Mafong EA, Kauvar AN, et al. Safety data of injectable nonanimal stabilized hyaluronic acid gel for soft tissue augmentation. Dermatol Surg 2002;28(6):491–4.

30. Raulin C, Greve B, Hartschuh W, et al. Exudative granulomatous reaction to hyaluronic acid (Hylaform). Contact Dermatitis 2000;43(3):178–9.

31. Fernandez-Acenero MJ, Zamora E, Borbujo J. Granulomatous foreign body reaction against hyaluronic acid: report of a case after lip augmentation. Dermatol Surg 2003;29(12):1225–6.

32. Lupton JR, Alster TS. Cutaneous hypersensitivity reaction to injectable hyaluronic acid gel. Dermatol Surg 2000;26(2):135–7.

33. Patel VJ, Bruck MC, Katz BE. Hypersensitivity reaction to hyaluronic acid with negative skin testing. Plast Reconstr Surg 2006;117(6):92e–4e.

34. Christensen L, Breiting V, Janssen M, et al. Adverse reactions to injectable soft tissue permanent fillers. Aesthetic Plast Surg 2005;29(1):34–48.

35. Rothschild LJ, Mancinelli RL. Life in extreme environments. Nature 2001;409(6823):1092–101.

36. Ceri H, Olson ME, Stremick C, et al. The Calgary Biofilm Device: new technology for rapid determination of antibiotic susceptibilities of bacterial biofilms. J Clin Microbiol 1999;37(6):1771–6.

37. Bjarnsholt T, Tolker-Nielsen T, Givskov M, et al. Detection of bacteria by fluorescence in situ hybridization in culture-negative soft tissue filler lesions. Dermatol Surg 2009;35(Suppl 2):1620–4.

38. Anwar H, Strap JL, Chen K, et al. Dynamic interactions of biofilms of mucoid *Pseudomonas aeruginosa* with tobramycin and piperacillin. Antimicrob Agents Chemother 1992;36(6):1208–14.

39. Dijkema SJ, van der Lei B, Kibbelaar RE. New-fill injections may induce late-onset foreign body granulomatous reaction. Plast Reconstr Surg 2005;115(5):76e–8e.

40. Christensen L. Normal and pathologic tissue reactions to soft tissue gel fillers. Dermatol Surg 2007;33(Suppl 2):S168–75.

41. Christensen LH. Host tissue interaction, fate, and risks of degradable and nondegradable gel fillers. Dermatol Surg 2009;35(Suppl 2):1612–9.

42. Yagi Y, Kato K, Murakami D, et al. Use of Aquamid as a filler for facial rejuvenation in orientals. J Plast Reconstr Aesthet Surg 2009;62(10):1245–9.

43. Weinkle SH, Bank DE, Boyd CM, et al. A multicenter, double-blind, randomized controlled study of the safety and effectiveness of Juvéderm injectable gel with and without lidocaine. J Cosmet Dermatol 2009;8(3):205–10.

44. Schiller D, Freeman JB, Mitchell JP, et al. A neural mechanism of first impressions. Nat Neurosci 2009;12(4):508–14.

45. Willis J, Todorov A. First impressions: making up your mind after a 100-ms exposure to a face. Psychol Sci 2006;17(7):592–8.

46. Bar M, Neta M, Linz H. Very first impressions. Emotion 2006;6(2):269–78.

47. Dayan S, Clark K, Ho AA. Altering first impressions after facial plastic surgery. Aesthetic Plast Surg 2004;28(5):301–6.

48. Dayan SH, Arkins JP, Gal TJ. Blinded evaluation of the effects of hyaluronic acid filler injections on first impressions. Dermatol Surg 2010;36(Suppl 3):1866–73.

49. Dayan SH, Lieberman ED, Thakkar NN, et al. Botulinum toxin a can positively impact first impression. Dermatol Surg 2008;34(Suppl 1):S40–7.

50. Moller AP. Developmental stability and fitness: a review. Am Nat 1997;149(5):916–32.

51. Thornhill R, Moller AP. Developmental stability, disease and medicine. Biol Rev Camb Philos Soc 1997;72(4):497–548.

52. Springer IN, Wannicke B, Warnke PH, et al. Facial attractiveness: visual impact of symmetry increases significantly towards the midline. Ann Plast Surg 2007;59(2):156–62.

53. Morris D. Body watching. Oxford (United Kingdom): Equinox Ltd; 1985.

54. Hickman L, Firestone AR, Beck FM, et al. Eye fixations when viewing faces. J Am Dent Assoc 2010;141(1):40–6.

55. Sarwer DB, Grossbart TA, Didie ER. Beauty and society. Semin Cutan Med Surg 2003;22(2):79–92.

56. Johnston VS. Mate choice decisions: the role of facial beauty. Trends Cogn Sci 2006;10(1):9–13.

SUGGESTED READINGS: ELLIS

Alcalay J, Alkalay R, Gat A, et al. Late-onset granulomatous reaction to Artecoll. Dermatol Surg 2003;29(8):859–62.

Carruthers J, Carruthers A, Tezel A, et al. Volumizing with 20-mg/ml smooth, highly cohesive, viscous hyaluronic acid filler and its role in facial rejuvenation therapy. Dermatol Surg 2010;36(Suppl 3):1886–92.

Cohen SR, Berner CF, Busso M, et al. Artefill: a long-lasting injectable wrinkle-filler material—summary of the U.S. Food and Drug Administration trials and a progress report on 4- to 5-year outcomes. Plast Reconstr Surg 2006;118(Suppl 3):64S–76S.

Dini L, Panzarini E, Micooli MA, et al. In vitro study of the interaction of polyalkylimide and polyvinyl alcohol hydrogels with cells. Tissue Cell 2005;37:479–87.

Eppley BL, Dadvand B. Injectable soft-tissue fillers: clinical overview. Plast Reconstr Surg 2006;118(4):98e–106e.

Formigli L, Zecchi S, Protopapa C, et al. Bio-Alcamid: an electron microscopic study after skin implantation. Plast Reconstr Surg 2004;113(3):1104–6.

Lemperle G, Morhenn V, Charrier U. Human histology and persistence of various injectable filler substances for soft tissue augmentation. Aesthetic Plast Surg 2003;27(3):354–67.

Lemperle G, Gauthier-Hazan N, Wolters M, et al. Foreign body granulomas after all injectable dermal fillers. Part I: possible causes. Plast Reconstr Surg 2009;123(6):1842–63.

Lemperle G, Knapp TR, Sadick NS, et al. Artefill permanent injectable for soft tissue augmentation: II. Indications and applications. Aesthetic Plast Surg 2010;34(3):273–86.

Manafi A, Emami A, Pooli AH, et al. Unacceptable results with an accepted soft tissue filler: polyacrylamide hydrogel. Aesthetic Plast Surg 2010;34:413–22.

Pacini S, Ruggiero M, Morucci G, et al. Bio-Alcamid: a novelty for reconstructive and cosmetic surgery. Ital J Anat Embryol 2002;107(3):209–14.

Ramires PA, Miccoli MA, Panzarini E, et al. In vitro and in vivo biocompatibility evaluation of a polyalkylimide hydrogel for soft tissue augmentation. J Biomed Mater Res B Appl Biomater 2005;72(2):230–8.

Romagnoli M, Belmontesi M. Hyaluronic acid-based fillers: theory and practice. Clin Dermatol 2008; 26(2):123–59.

Wolter TP, Pallua N. Removal of the permanent filler polyacrylamide hydrogel (Aquamid) is possible and easy even after several years. Plast Reconstr Surg 2010;126(3):138e–9e.

Fat Grafting: Discussion and Debate

Samuel Lam, MD[a],*, Thomas L. Tzikas, MD[b],*,
Mark Glasgold, MD[c],*

KEYWORDS

• Fat grafting • Alloplastic injectables • Autologous fat transfer • Skin rejuvenation

---

Fat Grafting

Samuel Lam, Thomas L. Tzikas, and Mark Glasgold address questions for discussion and debate:

1. With the increase in alloplastic injectables, is fat grafting dead?
2. Where do you think fat grafting fits in compared with the injectable implants?
3. Do you do grafting and injectables in some patients? If so, give examples.
4. How do you harvest and prepare fat for injection? Do you think that the process chosen impacts longevity of the grafts, and how long does fat last in your experience? What percentage usually takes in each site, and does the source or the site injected make a difference in this regard?
5. What areas of the face are most amenable to fat grafting, and how much fat should ideally be injected into each site?
6. *Analysis:* Over the past 5 years, how has your perspective evolved or what is the most important thing you have learned/observed regarding fat grafting?

With the increase in alloplastic injectables, is fat grafting dead?

LAM

The answer is absolutely not.[1] Fat grafting and fillers are both viable methods for facial rejuvenation and enhancement. Injectable fillers provide immediate gratification and minimal downtime for patients who are interested in using them. However, for someone with more substantive aging that requires multiple syringes, fat can provide more global restoration and be more durable than injectable fillers, which is discussed in the subsequent questions.

TZIKAS

On the contrary, fat grafting is more popular today and is performed by more physicians than at any other time. Injectable fillers have actually reinforced the idea that facial volume is the main consideration when attempting to restore youthful qualities to the aging face. Although injectable fillers are fairly straightforward and simple to perform, they alone cannot give the overall pan-facial improvement that fat grafting can. In my practice, facial fillers play an important role in introducing new patients to facial rejuvenation. Patients see an improvement in their facial

---

[a] Lam Facial Plastic Surgery Center, 6101 Chapel Hill Boulevard, Suite 101Plano, TX 75093, USA
[b] 526 Southeast 5th Avenue, Delray Beach, FL 33483, USA
[c] Glasgold Group Plastic Surgery, Highland Park Office, 31 River Road, Highland Park, NJ 08904, USA
* Corresponding authors.
E-mail addresses: drlam@lamfacialplastics.com; tzikasmd@gmail.com; info@glasgoldgroup.com

Facial Plast Surg Clin N Am 20 (2012) 265–278
doi:10.1016/j.fsc.2012.05.005
1064-7406/12/$ – see front matter © 2012 Elsevier Inc. All rights reserved.

appearance but, over the course of repeated injections and over a few years, many patients develop injection fatigue and desire a longer-lasting and more significant result. Fat grafting is the perfect logical next step in their rejuvenation and is almost always accompanied by other procedures, such as eyelid rejuvenation, laser skin treatment, or facelift surgery. Fat grafting provides a soft tissue layer of padding that aging patients are missing while improving the overall appearance and quality of the skin.

Injectable fillers are limited by volume and cost. It would be cost prohibitive to inject 10 or 20 syringes of a hyaluronic acid filler or calcium hydroxylapatite in a patient but this can easily be done with fat. The important distinction, however, is that fat is *not* an ideal filler for facial lines, such as nasolabial folds or glabellar creases. The method of injection is also different. Fat is injected in the deeper tissue planes and, therefore, requires a greater volume to augment an area.

There will most likely always be a place for alloplastic facial fillers because of their unique qualities, such as the superficial filling of facial lines. It is not that fat cannot fill these lines as well as the fillers, it can. Fat is presented to patients as a longer-lasting augmentation product and in areas, such as superficial facial folds in mobile regions, it is not better than the fillers with respect to longevity. Fat grafting, however, does give some long-term augmentation even in these areas but the percentage of fat taking is much less than in the less-superficial and less-mobile facial areas.

Where do you think fat grafting fits in compared with the injectable implants?

LAM

Alloplastic injectables can be a wonderful alternative to fat grafting, but each modality carries it owns merits, risks, and limitations. Fat grafting is a live graft that carries the risk of changes with weight gain or loss along with other metabolic changes that can occur with aging. Those who fluctuate in weight or are of prechildbearing age are on the higher-risk profile when working with fat grafting. In those patients, I prefer injectable fillers for their safety. In addition, younger patients or those who are overweight typically need fewer syringes of injectable product making it more cost beneficial to use off-the-shelf fillers. However, in someone aged more than 40 years, for example, who has ongoing hollowness of the face, I often need 40 to 50 mL of fat to achieve a remarkable global rejuvenation. I think each syringe of filler is equal to about 3 syringes of fat. Accordingly, it can become cost prohibitive to provide that degree of injectable product for a patient's face when harvested fat is free, so to speak. I also find that fat grafting provides a much softer look and feel to the face that may be partially attributable to stem cell effects (but I am not convinced entirely of this observation) but also because fat is softer in texture.

The limitation of fat grafting is that because it is a live graft it does not have 100% take, meaning that it is less predictable in any one area of the face than fillers would be. Therefore, if someone is interested in just having their cheeks augmented, it makes less sense for me to undertake a surgical procedure just to put some fat in the cheeks. I think it is more predictable to use fillers in this case. Also, with a permanent filler, like fat grafting, I think a person looks better when the permanent filler is blended evenly over multiple small areas rather than just stuck in one area of the face. Further, because fat is a very soft product it may not lift folds or creases or small skin divots as effectively as soft tissue fillers. I oftentimes use soft tissue fillers to augment my fat-grafting results when I see small areas that could use just a little bit more fat but where I think a fat graft would be unpredictable if the person went back under anesthesia and had a little more fat put in. I use the analogy of a bed to understand how I conceptualize the face for prospective patients. I think fat provides the mattress to the face; whereas fillers are the duvet that can fill in more surface problems. Neurotoxins and skin care can help with the outer sheets of the bed. In this way, I try to communicate with patients the benefits and limitations of fillers and fat grafting.

TZIKAS

In the first discussion I respond, in part, to this question. Additionally, one facial filler that has some of the attributes of fat grafting is poly-L-lactic acid. With repeated treatments, it results in

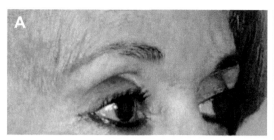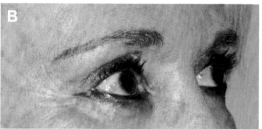

Fig. 1. Tzikas: (*A*) Hollow appearance of the orbital region following multiple eyelid surgeries. (*B*) Periorbital rejuvenation using fat grafting, 1.5 years.

a softness to facial areas, such as the midface, that resembles the appearance one can obtain with fat grafting. Poly-L-lactic acid has several limitations, however, most notably related to areas that it should not be injected because of the high incidence of nodules, which are not easily treated. Two such areas are the infraorbital region (**Fig. 1**A, B) and the lips. Fat grafting can be used in these areas with excellent outcomes, although more limited in the lips, and with an extremely low risk of complications.

Fat grafting should be thought of as a panfacial augmentation product because the face undergoes volume loss. Obviously, it is a more complex procedure than the injection of facial fillers and requires more training by the surgeon and with more recovery time for patients. Fat grafting requires that adequate volumes be injected to the face (at least 50 mL for the face) in a multilayered technique. My observations have been that the results seem to be softer over several years (**Fig. 2**A, B).

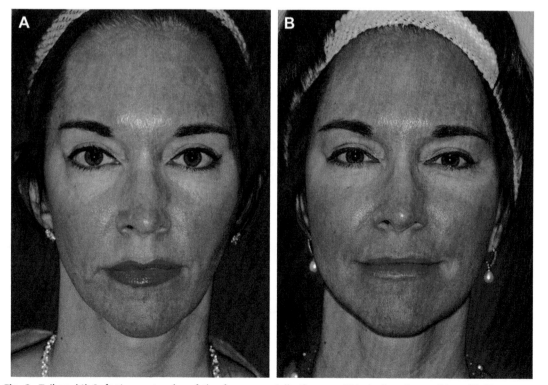

Fig. 2. Tzikas: (*A*) Soft tissue atrophy of the face, especially the mandible before fat grafting. (*B*) Three years following fat grafting to the face (88 mL). Note the overall softness and more youthful appearance.

Do you do grafting and injectables in some patients? If so, give examples

LAM

Yes, as elaborated in question 2 (*Where do you think fat grafting fits in compared with the injectable implants?*), I use fat grafting for specific patients and fillers for others and in some cases I use both. Let me clarify by being more succinct. I prefer fillers for those who are metabolically unstable to have safe fat grafting (too young or with fluctuating weight profiles); those who want just a little area of the face managed, like the cheek, lips, or nasolabial grooves; those who have limited downtime or must be looking good for an upcoming event that is soon; those who are afraid of fat grafting or do not understand it; those who cannot afford to have fat grafting but just want a little injectable filler (I like to say that is like buying a little bit of fat grafting at a time); those who simply do not have enough donor fat to do sufficient work; those who have had fat grafting and would like a touch up or to maintain their result against further aging; and those who are unsafe surgical candidates for whatever reason.

For me, fat grafting is suggested for those individuals who want the best global, durable, and beautiful results and can afford to undergo the procedure in terms of cost, recovery, and safety (as described previously). I like to look at fat grafting as the Ferrari of results because I really do not think facial fillers can get close to the beauty and softness of a fat-grafting result when it is done well and artistically by an experienced practitioner of this art and science.

TZIKAS

Yes, fat grafting is often used for augmenting the face as a standalone procedure or it can be used to augment the midface and upper face when combined with several types of surgeries, such as fractional CO_2 laser resurfacing, blepharoplasty, facelift, or even rhinoplasty. On many occasions, the fine perioral lines are treated with microdroplet Silikon-1000 (Alcon Labs, Fort Worth, TX, USA) injections at the same time. This treatment is an off-label Food and Drug Administration (FDA) use of this product but has been rewarding for this application in my practice. Other fillers, such as hyaluronic acids or calcium hydroxylapatite, are sometimes used in conjunction with fat to fill in the superficial portion of a nasolabial or glabellar fold for which fat does not correct as well.

A cost-effective procedure that has become popular in my older patient population is a combination of moderate volume (20–30 mL) midfacial and upper-facial fat grafting with a silicone injection to the perioral rhytids and fractional CO_2 laser resurfacing of the face. This procedure provides correction of the 2 major components of facial aging, volume loss in the midface and facial rhytids caused by environmental factors, with a short recovery time of 7 to 10 days.

How do you harvest and prepare fat for injection? Do you think that the process chosen impacts longevity of the grafts, and how long does fat last in your experience? What percentage usually takes in each site, and does the source or the site injected make a difference in this regard?

LAM

I harvest my fat by hand (as opposed to machine) using 10-mL syringes with 1 to 3 mL of negative pressure. I then centrifuge the fat for 3 minutes at 3000 rpm, decant the supranatant and infranatant, further wick off the supranatant, and then transfer the fat into 1-mL Luer-Lok (BD Medical, Franklin Lakes, NJ, USA) syringes outfitted with 1.2-mm or 0.9-mm Tulip injection cannulas (Tulip Medical Products, San Diego, California) (**Fig. 3**). I do not necessarily think that one processing method is superior to another. I trained with a Japanese surgeon in Tokyo who washed and

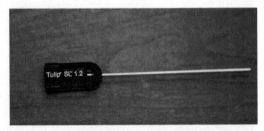

Fig. 3. Lam: This is image is a close-up of the 1.2-mm cannula manufactured by Tulip Medical Products, which is used as the workhorse injector for the face and hands. Additionally, a 0.9-mm wide cannula is used selectively for the temple region.

filtered his fat and has shown tremendous longevity of a decade and more. I think that the processing element has been overemphasized. I think it is important to find a surgeon with a mature practice who demonstrates longevity and then to follow that technique rather than trying to reinvent the wheel when it comes to processing methodology. I learned my method from Mark Glasgold who has shown good longevity with his fat results. However, I have matured my thinking of the artistic element of how to inject the fat to create results that are uniquely my own.

I think that fat grafting is truly permanent (**Fig. 4**). I have likened a fat transplant result to a hair transplant. With a hair transplant, you see a result that matures over a period of 1 to 2 years as neovascularization starts to take place. I have carefully studied my results over the years and have seen a bell curve whereby the fat gets better over the first 1 to 2 years and there is a slight decline year by year thereafter. This bell curve is similar to a hair transplant in which ongoing hair loss of non-transplanted hair represents further aging. The transplanted fat is durable like a hair graft. However, the remaining fat of the face continues to be lost as one ages, just as the natural untransplanted hairs on the head follow the same pathway of loss. Accordingly, the result is permanent minus ongoing aging. I know twins, one of whom is about 5 years out from fat grafting. Although the one I operated on has aged more than 5 years, she still looks remarkably younger than her sister. I like to use the analogy of a glass of water that continues to empty despite having been filled up one time (ie, the glass of water is always fuller than it would have been if it had never been filled but it has slowly gone down with further time).

In terms of how much percentage of fat grafting takes, I do not have a solid scientific answer. I think there is definitely some degree of variability as shown in a study that Dr Glasgold has elegantly performed. However, I think that if enough areas of the face are augmented with fat, then the global outcome can still be amazing despite any one area not being perfect. I think that most fat-grafting surgeons would agree that the perioral area is less than ideal in terms of take. Despite some concerns regarding smokers and older individuals, I have seen pretty good take that is uniform despite these limitations.

TZIKAS

The patients' donor areas of fat excess are evaluated for quality and possible limitations caused by the lack of sufficient quantity or a previous site of liposuction. Multiple donor areas are marked with the patient in the standing position. It is important to obtain fat from multiple sites, especially in thin patients, so that the potential for donor deformities from too much fat extraction from one location is limited. The best quality donor fat in most patients is found in the lateral thighs because of the compactness of the adipocytes, but the medial thighs, the upper hips, the lower abdomen, and sometimes the medial knees are also used. The procedure is usually performed using conscious intravenous sedation with local nerve blocks and local anesthetic soft tissue infiltration (1% lidocaine with 1:100,000 epinephrine) in the face. A semitumescent local infiltration is performed in the donor areas using a mixture of 50 mL of 1% lidocaine, 1 mL of 1:1000 epinephrine, and 12.5 mL sodium bicarbonate in 1 L of lactated ringers solution. The anesthetic fluid is injected through entry sites made with a #11 blade first into the deep fat followed by the more superficial layer using 20-mL syringes and multi-holed fine infiltrating cannulas. This process results in some volume expansion of the adipocytes, which must be taken into account during facial infiltration. It is important to wait at least 15 minutes for the local epinephrine effect to occur before fat harvesting. The quality and quantity of harvested fat will be significantly enhanced after this waiting period. For fat harvesting, 2.4-mm multi-holed aspirating cannulas (Tulip Medical Products, San Diego, CA, USA) attached to a 10-mL syringe are used. Approximately 2 mL of lactated ringers solution is placed in each syringe before harvesting, and a minimal negative volume pressure on the syringe is used, usually 2 to 3 mL, to limit the trauma to the harvested fat. The amount of fat and fluid aspirated during harvesting is measured to remove equal amounts from the contralateral side. The donor access sites are closed with a 5-0 fast-absorbing suture, and the area is dressed with a light pressure dressing.

The fat is centrifuged for 4 minutes at 3000 rpm in the 10-mL syringes, which results in 3 distinct layers. The fat for injection should not contain any significant amount of blood because blood will stimulate macrophage activity in the recipient site and may decrease fat survival. The fatty layer is separated from the other layers by decanting the fluid from the syringes. The usable fat is ultimately transferred into 1-mL syringes, which are then used for the injection of fat into the face.

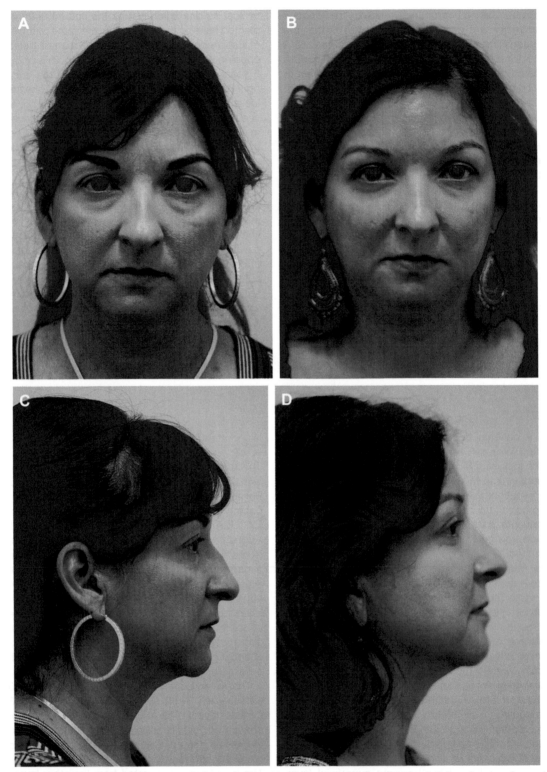

Fig. 4. Lam: This 46-year-old woman is shown before (*A, C*) and 1 year after (*B, D*) a full-face fat transfer and rhinoplasty with good aesthetic improvement and rejuvenation.

Fat grafting, when done properly, will last several years and is considered, in my opinion, to be permanent. The process does not have to be performed exactly as described previously. When I first started injecting fat in 1995, I was aspirating fat with larger cannulas and washing the fat through a strainer. Results were also good with that particular technique. I think as long as the surgeon does not overtraumatize the fat graft or allow it to desiccate by being exposed to room air, there is good viability. The volume of fat injected into the face (50–80 mL) and the technique of multilayered injection are also important.

It is difficult to assess the percentage of fat that takes after injection. The regions of the face injected will have a differing viability of fat. Experience has shown that fat grafts are less predictable and have overall less survival in mobile areas, such as the lips and the perioral regions. Fat grafts that are placed in the perioral region are viable, but the result is less predictable because of the mobility associated with the area. This results in shearing forces, which limit the angiogenesis to the graft. Repeat treatments with frozen fat or other filler materials are used, especially in the lips and marionette regions. The popular myth that autologous fat grafting is a temporary filler is primarily a result of surgeons injecting fat into mostly mobile areas, such as the lips or nasolabial grooves; using poor technique; and not injecting adequate volumes. This misconception is a hurdle the clinician must overcome when dealing with patients questioning the viability of fat grafting and long-term results.

There is also variability with the survival of fat between patients. Patients aged younger than 60 years who are nonsmokers and have no chronic diseases tend to retain a greater percentage of fat; however, all patients retain fat. The results are subtler than facelift or rhinoplasty surgery, and quality preprocedure and postprocedure photography is essential to review with patients.

What areas of the face are most amenable to fat grafting, and how much fat should ideally be injected into each site?

LAM

I think almost every part of the face is amenable to fat grafting: temples, brows, upper eyelid, lower eyelid, nasojugal groove, anterior cheek, lateral cheek, buccal, subzygomatic region, mandible, postjowl, prejowl, anterior chin, canine fossa, and nasolabial groove. How much fat to place into each area is truly a question of technique and artistry. In Dr Glasgold's and my book, *Complementary Fat Grafting*,[1] we outlined some basic amounts of fat that are suggested for transplantation. Over the years, I have made some modifications by ongoing studies of my results. I think it is important that a surgeon have a firm grasp on the technical basics of fat transfer and then over time adapt those quantities as one reviews his or her results. In general, I like to use about 3 mL of fat into each lower eyelid, about 0.1 to 0.5 mL into the lateral canthus, about 1 to 2 mL into the brow/upper eyelid complex, about 1 to 2 mL into the anterior cheek, about 1 to 2 mL into the lateral cheek, about 0 to 5 mL into the buccal area, about 2 to 3 mL into the prejowl region, and about 2 to 4 mL into the anterior chin. These numbers refer to one side of the face only and are truly just a range that I use but vary based on a person's facial shape, aging, and so forth.

TZIKAS

As mentioned previously, the most successful areas of fat grafting are in the more static regions of the face, such as the tear trough deformity, the midface, the upper malar region, the jawline, the temporal fossa, the mandible, and the lateral eyebrow. Fat grafts that are placed in the perioral region are viable, but the result is less predictable because of the mobility associated with the area.

Fat infiltration of the face begins by making skin puncture sites at strategic locations using an 18-gauge NoKor needle (BD Medical, Franklin Lakes, NJ, USA). The facial access sites are closed for 24 hours with steristrips (3M, Mapelwood, MN, USA) and usually heal without a visible mark. Generally, 0.9-mm and 1.2-mm cannulas (Tulip Medical Products, San Diego, CA, USA) are attached to 1-mL syringes filled with the fat grafts and are used to inject the fat. The 1-mL syringes allow for a smoother transfer of fat grafts while minimizing force. The infiltration is first performed in the deepest tissue layer (usually at the supraperiosteal level) and along the facial musculature and then followed by more superficial layers. The injection of fat is performed only on withdrawal of the cannula in linear tracts, ultimately creating a weaving pattern.

There is no ideal volume of fat that should be injected to each region of the face. This amount varies in all patients and is most closely related to the age of the patient and the overall elasticity of the skin. The most delicate infiltration is in the infraorbital region where injection is mostly submuscular but superficial to the orbital septum and always in a retrograde fashion. Some fat infiltration is performed in the subcutaneous layer using only small quantities of fat (usually between 0.025–0.05 mL per tunnel) to prevent clumping. It usually requires approximately 10 to 20 passes to empty a 1-mL syringe of fat in most parts of the face; but in the infraorbital area, even less fat is injected per pass. Fat infiltration along the infraorbital rim is mostly injected from an inferior to superior position. The nasojugal and tear trough regions are also infiltrated from an inferior midmalar position injecting superiorly. The fat is injected in small *noncontinuous* amounts rather than one long strand. A long continuous injection of fat in the infraorbital region can result in elevated abnormalities that are visible through the thin skin and can be challenging to treat. Some fat is also injected from a lateral orbital skin entry site from which injection can also be performed to the lateral eyebrow, the anterior and inferior temple, and the main malar and submalar regions. The volume of fat injected varies for all individuals; but along the infraorbital rim and tear trough regions, the volume should generally be limited to approximately 2 mL.

The overall malar region, however, can accept 7 to 20 mL of fat spread over a wide area. It is important to feather the fat into adjacent aesthetic zones by injecting the anterior temporal region and the lateral eyebrow. This practice creates a soft transition when performing midface augmentation. The success of the technique depends on the injection of only small amounts of fat into many multilayered tunnels, which leads to improved revascularization and survival of the graft. It is also important not to overfill the anterior malar and infraorbital region because this will create excessive fullness and skin wrinkling when smiling. Fat should be tapered as the injection is continued toward the eyelid, so a resultant ledge of fat or sunken eye appearance can be avoided. The infiltration of fat is a diffuse process following the natural bony and soft tissue facial architecture of the patient, and volumes injected for the whole face can vary from 50 to more than 100 mL.

Analysis: Over the past 5 years, how has your perspective evolved or what is the most important thing you have learned/observed regarding fat grafting?

LAM

Most of my ideas have already been expressed in the previous discussions. However, here are the most important things that I have learned over the past 5 years:

1. Fat grafting evolves over time and is truly a live graft. Choosing safe patients is predicated on finding someone who does not have a high-risk profile: very young or with fluctuating weight issues. Also, because fat grafting actually improves in most cases over 1 to 2 years, I try to avoid touching up or messing with my fat results for at least 1 year.
2. Fat grafting is an artistic endeavor in which areas of the face can be augmented not only to create a more youthful face but a more balanced one. When someone is very gaunt,

putting fat into the buccal area can help gently widen the face to create a more oval face. In contrast, someone who is wider or heavier can be made to seem less heavy by filling more into the anterior chin and into the upper central cheek region.

3. Fat grafting can be combined with fillers effectively to create the most optimal results, with fat grafting providing the foundation for the face and fillers to augment small areas of the face that would benefit from small touch-ups.
4. Like anything, patient communication, frequent follow-up, and photographic review help to establish appropriate expectations and to review the benefits with patients who may forget how they used to look over time. These elements are important to a successful practice.

TZIKAS

One of the key aspects of my technique that has changed over the past 5 years is related to the overall volume of fat that is injected. Although I still inject large volumes to the face, it is extremely rare that this total would exceed 100 mL for the face. I find that volumes between 50 to 80 mL result in

less facial edema while maintaining a good long-term result.

The time that fat is centrifuged has increased to about 4 minutes. I find that the concentration of the fat in the syringe is more compact and, therefore, allows for more predictable results. Too much oil

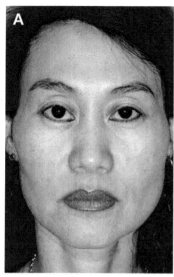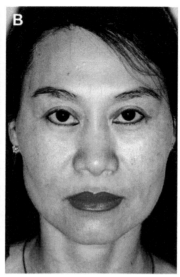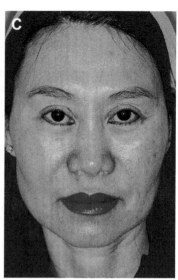

Fig. 5. Tzikas: (*A*) Preoperative significant bony facial asymmetry and hollowing of the temples. (*B*) Twenty-six months following fat grafting (66 mL) to the face and upper blepharoplasty. Note the better symmetry of the overall face. (*C*) Persistent results 7.5 years after the procedure.

or liquid mixed with the fat results in less adequate volume restoration and a great degree of unpredictability.

I have learned to be more conservative with the volume injected in the infraorbital region. I use the smallest cannulas possible (0.7 or 0.9 mm) and always try to undercorrect in this area. Injecting small aliquots of noncontinuous fat will give the best results. Fat clumping from overinjection in this area is difficult to correct and should be avoided.

Another important aspect of the art of fat grafting to the face is to review patients' facial photos from previous decades. This practice is a valuable teaching tool for both the surgeon and the patients. This practice gives the surgeon an idea of the type of face the patients had in their youth and prevents the desire to radically alter their proportions. It also stresses the importance of volume depletion with facial aging to patients.

Soft tissue augmentation with fat grafting is technique dependent with a high learning curve. The surgeon must master a precise minimally traumatic harvesting, preparation, and infiltration technique using a diffuse multilayering method of fat infiltration, which follows the patient's facial contour. The main benefit of fat is that it is a natural filler, which can augment all areas of a face.

GLASGOLD

Relating to the question of technique evolution, I wonder if our tendency as surgeons to be primarily technique oriented dictates the type of

Autologous fat grafting results can be extremely satisfying for both patients and the surgeon as long as the expectations are realistic. A small amount of fat grafted into multiple tunnels undergoes revascularization and becomes incorporated into normal subcutaneous tissue. Grafted fat feels like normal soft tissue to the touch and cannot be palpated like other facial implants. Results at 5 or 6 months usually persist for many years, although normal soft tissue volume loss continues with natural aging. Grafted fat will also fluctuate in size with general weight loss or weight gain. There is some individual patient variability noted with younger patients retaining a greater percentage of fat using smaller volumes, which is most likely because of the better vascularity and tissue elasticity in younger patients.

Autologous fat grafting results are subtle yet significant, with the face appearing softer, healthier, and more youthful without having the operated look. The resultant facial contour has a natural appearance with a gentle transition between one facial zone and the next. The fat-infiltration technique is an artistic 3-dimensional (3D) procedure, and patient outcomes improve with greater experience by the surgeon. Once the technique is mastered, results are long-term and predictable and can complement most other facial surgical procedures (**Fig. 5**A–C).

results we produce or should the result we are trying to achieve dictate the techniques we choose to use?

This question is at the heart of my evolution with the technique of autologous fat transfer. Facial rejuvenation surgery, when I entered the field in the mid 1990s, was a specialty that was experiencing tremendous growth and change in the procedures we had to evaluate and learn. Endoscopic brow lifting was being taught at hands-on courses for the first time and every month a new variation of midface lifting was being presented. I would go to meetings and become overwhelmed with all of the techniques I did not know and had to learn. There was the great CO_2 laser debate (Sharplan [Sharplan Lasers, Inc., Allendale, NJ, USA] vs coherent) and the debate of deep-plane facelift versus superficial musculo-aponeurotic system facelift still goes on today.

With the endless enthusiasm of youth, I went through many excruciating learning curves trying techniques. I developed into a surgeon with an extensive surgical toolbox looking to put these tools to practical use. I was a technician not engaged in the pursuit of facial rejuvenation but focused on performing facial plastic surgery procedures. In 1998, I took a fat-transfer course with Dr Sydney Coleman. I learned almost nothing about the actual technique of fat grafting, but I was transformed by his vision of facial rejuvenation based on volume replacement.

Only recently has there been widespread acceptance of volume replacement as a fundamental part of the facial rejuvenation paradigm and autologous fat transfer as a fundamental technique for achieving volume.[2] It has been gratifying that volume replacement has now become the centerpiece for many of our facial-rejuvenation meetings.[3] There are 2 main issues that I think are central to any discussion of autologous fat transfer: How do we most precisely delineate the locations where volume is placed to maximize facial rejuvenation? How do we increase the predictability of the technique?

When I first became interested in autologous fat grafting, the procedure was being presented as an exacting artistic endeavor that was not easily learned. My evolution with the technique taught me that fat grafting for facial rejuvenation could be presented as a reproducible algorithmic procedure that could produce consistent and complication-free results. With the help of Dr Robert Glasgold and Dr Samuel Lam, the book, *Complementary Fat Grafting*,[1] presented an approach that can be taught and implemented in a concise manner. We presented the concept of a volumetric foundation whereby quantified amounts of fat are placed in precise locations on the face defined by bone or surface landmarks (**Fig. 6**). The volumetric foundation is a cookbook-type recipe that can be used on almost all faces and becomes the basis of the learning curve for the new surgeon.

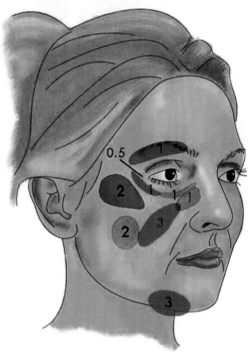

VOLUMETRIC FOUNDATION
(Fat Volumes, 14.5 cc/side)

Fig. 6. Glasgold: Volumetric foundation.

Complementary fat grafting was the initial step in evolving our understanding of where to place volume. We have become convinced that the key to facial rejuvenation lies in understanding that the aging appearance occurs primarily because of the development of facial shadows in patterns, which we recognize at a subconscious level. For the most part, these shadows occur as a result of volume loss, skin re-draping, and facial retaining ligaments.[4] Robert and I have been working to describe these patterns in significant detail and they create a precise blueprint for the addition of volume to faces.[5]

Two common areas, the midface and the jawline, will demonstrate this idea. The hollow of the inferior orbital rim creates a shadow that demarcates the transition in an aging face between the lower eyelid and the cheek. The midface depression results from the malar septum and creates a midfacial shadow that runs parallel to the nasolabial fold (**Fig. 7**). These shadows are the critical shadows that the artist uses to convey aging in a drawing. If we fill the hollows and create a midface that has no distinction between the cheek and the lower lid and a unified midface highlight, we create a naturally appearing midface (**Fig. 8**). In the lower face, a youthful jawline appears as a straight line

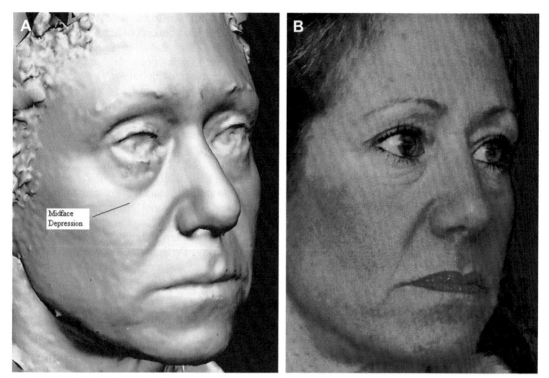

Fig. 7. Glasgold: Significant shadows of aging of the midface: (A) 3D rendering and (B) photograph.

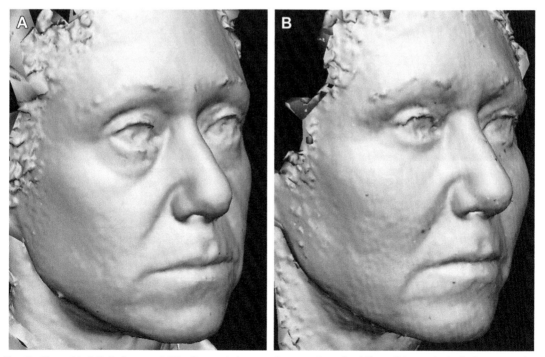

Fig. 8. Glasgold: (A) Before and (B) after autologous fat transfer of midface (3D rendering) demonstrating shadows converted to highlights.

between shadow below and light above.[6] The jowl breaks up this straight line to create a pattern of shadow, highlight, and shadow (**Fig. 9**). Sometimes a facelift will fail to restore the youthful appearance because what is really necessary is volume in the prejowl sulcus and lateral jawline.[7]

If we fill in hollows and turn the shadows of aging to highlights, we make the face look younger (**Fig. 10**). Unfortunately, today, volume replacement has at times become about quantity not subtlety. Celebrities who have had so much volume added that their appearance is radically altered are in all of the tabloids and scare our patients. The amount of volume necessary for improvement is just the amount needed to make this transition from shadow to highlight and is usually much less than most of us think. The role of greater volume is to change the shape of the face, which is a secondary characteristic of youth and beauty. The aging process makes faces seem more rectangular, the jowls square off the base while the cheeks deflate; restoring the heart shape to a female face is attractive, youthful, and feminine appearing. Our current work is focused on developing an easily understood algorithmic approach to treating the hollows that cause the shadows of facial aging and will allow surgeons

to understand how to recreate a youthful appearance rather than balloon heads.

Early on, the ability to achieve long-lasting results with autologous fat grafting was the primary subject of debate. Poor technique that led to lumps of fat that had to be removed was part of my technical learning curve. Excising these lumps demonstrated to me that it was transferred fat that was surviving.[8] I have documented in my practice results lasting for as long as 8 years, but I have also had patients with multiple transfers that have been unable to produce a lasting result. Because patients continue to lose facial volume over time, it is almost impossible to determine what is happening to the transferred fat.

The real problem with autologous fat transfer is predictability. Dr Robert Glasgold and Dr Jason Meier studied our long-term (>1 year) results of fat grafting using 3D photographic technology and showed that in our relatively expert hands fat grafting was predictably unpredictable.[9] At the same time, patient satisfaction with the results was high and only about 20% of the patients had a touch-up. This is consistent with my clinical experience over many years. The variables that need to be examined are harvesting technique and donor site, processing methods, injection

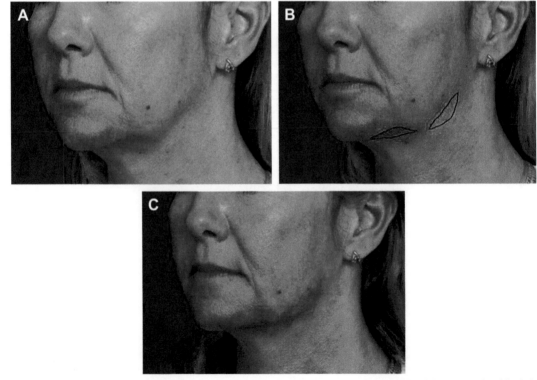

Fig. 9. Glasgold: (*A*) Jowl defined by shadow of prejowl sulcus and lateral mandible, (*B*) areas to be filled, (*C*) after volume rejuvenation of jawline.

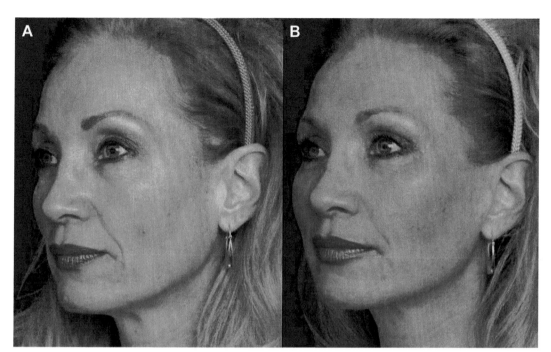

Fig. 10. Glasgold: (*A*) Before and (*B*) after autologous fat transfer.

technique, and the limitless patient variables that plague the results of all of our surgeries.

I intuitively harvest from the areas that patients feel are the most diet-resistant fat. It is fairly well accepted that harvesting and injection should be done with an emphasis on not traumatizing the fat, particularly with high suction. I prefer to use hand suction with a 10-mL syringe for harvesting. For injection, I use 1-mL syringes with a 9-mm diameter cannula and use a widespread fanning technique at multiple tissue depths.

I think that the greatest gains in predictability will come from improved processing techniques. Until recently, I centrifuged the fat. PureGraft is a membrane filtration system manufactured by Cytori Therapeutics (San Diego, CA, USA) that is easy to use and produces a quality of fat that cannot be achieved with any other processing technique. Fat processing with centrifugation, in my experience, will produce about a 40% yield of fat that can be injected. Centrifuged fat is noticeably contaminated with free fatty acids and

blood. PureGraft processing produces less fat for injection, yielding about 20% to 25% of the harvested fat. However, the PureGraft fat is much thicker and has no visible contamination with free fatty acids or blood components. When injected, it creates a much greater structural effect than centrifuged fat, and I am currently performing minimal overcorrection in my procedures. We are currently doing a 3D photographic long-term volumetric study to see if PureGraft processing will improve the predictability of the procedure.

The most exciting development in the area of fat transfer is the ability to isolate adipose-derived stem cells from fat within a single procedure using StemSource (Celution in Europe) equipment (Cytori Therapeutics, San Diego, CA, USA). The stem cells can then be added to the fat graft. This work is currently experimental[10] but it holds tremendous promise in both improving the take of fat grafts and possibly supercharging the skin rejuvenation that we commonly see after fat-grafting procedures.

REFERENCES

1. Lam S, Glasgold M, Glasgold R. Complementary fat grafting. Philadelphia: Lippincott, Williams & Wilkins; 2007.
2. Glasgold MJ, Lam SM, Glasgold RA. Complementary fat grafting. In: Papel I, editor. Facial plastic and reconstructive surgery. 3rd edition. New York: Thieme; 2008.
3. Rejuvenation of the aging face, AAFPRS, 1/19–23, San Diego (CA); 2011.
4. Donath AS, Glasgold RA, Glasgold MJ. Volume loss versus gravity: new concepts in facial aging. Curr Opin Otolaryngol Head Neck Surg 2007;15: 238–43.

5. Glasgold MJ, Glasgold RA, Lam SM. Volume restoration and facial aesthetics. Facial Plast Surg Clin North Am 2008;16(4):435–42.

6. Glasgold M, Lam SM, Glasgold R. Volumetric rejuvenation of the periorbital region. Facial Plast Surg 2010;26(3):252–9.

7. Glasgold M, Lam S, Glasgold R. Autologous fat grafting for cosmetic enhancement of the perioral region. Facial Plast Surg Clin North Am 2007;15:461–70.

8. Lam SM, Glasgold RA, Glasgold MJ. Limitations, complications, and long-term sequelae of fat transfer. Facial Plast Surg Clin North Am 2008; 16(4):391–9.

9. Meier JM, Glasgold RA, Glasgold MJ. Autologous fat grafting: long term evidence of its efficacy in mid-facial rejuvenation. Arch Facial Plast Surg 2009; 11(1):24–8.

10. Rigotti G, Marchi A, Galiè M, et al. Clinical treatment of radiotherapy tissue damage by lipoaspirate transplant: a healing process mediated by adipose-derived adult stem cells. Plast Reconstr Surg 2007;119(5):1409–22 [discussion: 1423–4].

Facelift
Panel Discussion, Controversies, and Techniques

E. Gaylon McCollough, MD[a],*, Stephen Perkins, MD[b],
J. Regan Thomas, MD[c]

KEYWORDS

- Facelift • Cosmetic surgery • Surgery techniques • Facelift candidate • Facelift results
- Minimally invasive surgery • Facial surgery mastery

Facelift Panel Discussion

Gaylon McCollough, Stephen Perkins, and J. Regan Thomas address questions for discussion and debate:

1. Who is not a candidate for facelift?

2. Of the various approaches to facelift, do any truly add advantages to an SMAS technique (ie, deep plane facelift)?

3. What techniques are most effective in managing the neckline in face-lifting and in what sequence should these be performed?

4. Which, if any, face-lifting techniques have been proved to provide the longest lasting result?

5. To start, develop, and maintain a busy face-lifting practice, is it necessary or even beneficial to offer some sort of minimalist facelift procedure or even a noninvasive substitute procedure?

6. *Analysis:* Over the past 5 years, how has your technique or approach changed, or what is the most important thing you have learned in performing facelifts?

Stephen Perkins presents videos of his facelift technique: Sequential Submental Excision and Plication of Subplatysmal Fat and Platysma; Undermining post auricular neck skin flap in rhytidectomy; Submentalplasty in Rhytidectomy; SMAS imbrication; and Submental and Jowl Liposuction in Rhytidectomy. Available at: http://www.facialplastic.theclinics.com

Who is not a candidate for facelift?

McCOLLOUGH

Patients who are not in good physical and/or mental health or those who present to a facial plastic surgeon with unrealistic expectations are not good candidates for any appearance-

---

[a] McCollough Plastic Surgery Clinic, 350 Cypress Bend Drive, PO Box 4249, Gulf Shores, AL 36547, USA
[b] Meridian Plastic Surgeons, 170 West 106th Street, Indianapolis, IN 46290, USA
[c] Department of Otolaryngology, Eye and Ear Institute, University of Illinois at Chicago, 1855 West Taylor, 3rd Floor, Chicago, IL 60612, USA
* Corresponding author.
E-mail addresses: drmccollough@mcculloughinstitute.com; sperkski@gmail.com; thomasrj@uic.edu

Facial Plast Surg Clin N Am 20 (2012) 279–325
doi:10.1016/j.fsc.2012.02.001
1064-7406/12/$ – see front matter © 2012 Published by Elsevier Inc

altering surgery. On a more global scale, a patient whose face requires more—or less—than what a "one-size-fits-all" facelift can provide is not a candidate for such a procedure...except in certain circumstances.

Some lifestyle habits affect eligibility for certain types of facelifts and ancillary procedures. Patients who use nicotine in any form are not good candidates for procedures that require extensive skin undermining. However, nicotine use should not automatically disqualify patients from rejuvenation procedures. Short flaps (ie, minimal skin elevation in the appropriate anatomic regions) with suspension of the underlying superficial muscular aponeurotic system (SMAS) and

minimal tension on the skin may be an acceptable alternative, as long as the patient understands that by limiting the procedure the overall result will be compromised.

Nicotine users must also understand that flap necrosis and unsightly scars are known risks and must be willing to accept them, in advance of surgery. In all cases, the surgeon should stress abstinence from nicotine for a minimum of 2 weeks before, and after, surgery. Oral niacin (in doses that produce a flush 4 times daily) and topical nitroglycerine paste applied over the undermined areas may be beneficial, especially should the blood supply to *any* facial flap become questionable.

THOMAS

The ideal candidate for a facelift would be an individual whose facial appearance is characterized best by a strong angular bony skeleton with a normal or high positioned hyoid complex. The patient should be at near ideal weight with minimal facial and submental fat and appropriate facial skin elasticity. The ideal patient would have relatively

smooth non-sun-damaged skin and be without deep rhytids. Certainly the ideal patient would be a healthy individual without systemic disease and would be psychologically realistic and well motivated, whose goal for surgery is improvement and not perfection. Thus the patient who is *not* an ideal candidate for facelift would be a patient who

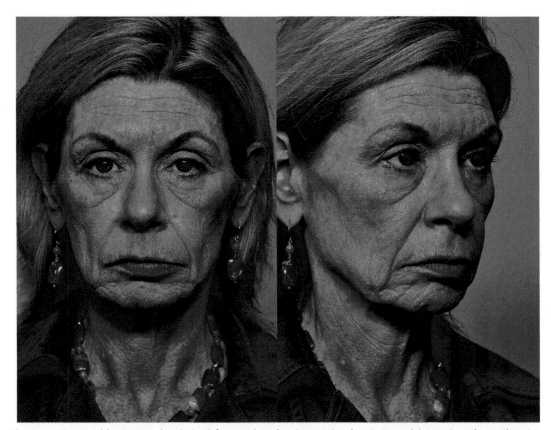

Fig. 1. A 57-year-old woman who desired face and neck rejuvenation but is a recalcitrant 2-pack-per-day cigarette smoker.

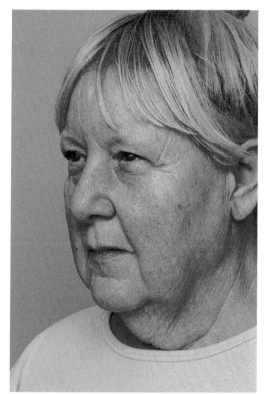

Fig. 2. A 60-year-old woman who is markedly over-weight and recently underwent bariatric surgery who desires a neck-lift. At present, this obese patient is not a candidate for facelift surgery until she loses her proposed weight.

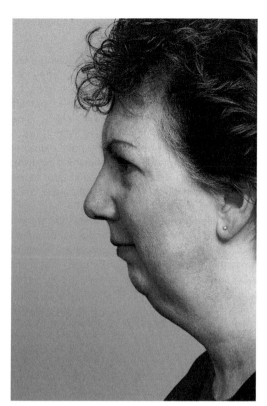

Fig. 3. A 57-year-old preoperative facelift patient with microgenia and a very low hyoid is a poor candidate for facelift surgery.

does not fulfill these ideal patient characteristics in a significant manner. Also note that it is important that the patient stop taking medications that would have an anticoagulant effect, including aspirin or nonsteroidal antiinflammatory drugs and vitamin E. Smoking has been demonstrated to impede healing, and the patient should quit smoking for at least 3 to 6 months before surgery.

PERKINS

Individuals who are not candidates for facelift include

- Active smokers (**Fig. 1**)
- Patients who could be in the middle of a life-changing situation (ie, divorce) or who are emotionally unstable and unrealistic and feel that the surgery will improve their life situation
- Obese patients, particularly those who are not controlling their weight and have large fluctuations or plan a significant weight loss in the next 3 to 6 months following surgery (**Fig. 2**)
- Patients unable to tolerate either deep sedation or general anesthesia or who are medically not cleared for surgery for cardiac or other reasons
- Patients who have active vasculitis or auto-immune diseases specifically related to the facial skin, such as facial scleroderma
- Patients on chemotherapy or a chemothera-peutic type medication controlling their autoimmune disease
- Patients with a history of full course radia-tion to the preauricular and infra-auricular neck skin, that is, those who have compro-mised vascularity due to chronic radiation or long-term previous chronic radiation exposure

The additional category of poor candidates for facelift should also be noted:

- Patients with a low hyoid, producing a very obtuse cervicomental angle, may not achieve a result or one that they expect to obtain. This is true in addition to patients who have markedly weak chins, small mandibles, or thick heavy skin (**Figs. 3 and 4**). Those patients who have extremely ptotic submandibular glands may be disappointed in their neckline result after facelift because of these glands becoming more obvious.
- Patients with very deep nasolabial grooves and prominent cheek mounds and folds are not ideal for this procedure because the facelift procedure itself does not adequately correct this and the patient may well feel that this is what a facelift does when it, in fact, does not improve that region (see **Figs. 2 and 3**).

A facelift can safely be performed on patients who are poor candidates as long as structural augmentation is added and/or they are completely realistic and are shown the results that are obtainable with their anatomy before the surgery.

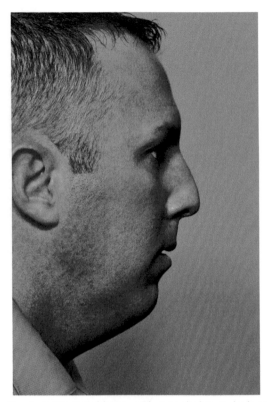

Fig. 4. A 42-year-old man with a weak chin and a low hyoid desires a "sharp" neckline. He remains a poor candidate for significant improvement in his neck from facelift surgery.

Of the various approaches to facelift, do any truly add advantages to an SMAS technique (ie, deep plane facelift)?

McCOLLOUGH

The so-called deep plane facelift has created confusion within plastic surgical circles, for it is, simply, an extension of the same SMAS suspension procedures that many facial plastic surgeons have been performing since the late 1970s. The principle difference in the most well-known version of the technique is that the sub-SMAS dissection is carried farther into the cheek and neck than was described in articles published by this author, and others, in the early 1980s.

In all primary lifts, and in every subsequent lift in which it is possible to raise an SMAS flap, the SMAS should be freed beyond the anterior border of the parotid gland and far enough anteriorly and inferiorly to allow for upward and backward movement of the cheek, lower face, and neck (refer to **Fig. 36** in the section "Facelift Approaches and Techniques from the Masters").

When the posterior margin of the newly developed SMAS flap is tugged on with surgical forceps, the surgeon should witness upward and backward movement of the cheek and neck tissues. In my experience, any dissection beyond this point of mobilization is fruitless and increases the risk of injury to branches of the facial nerve.

THOMAS

Having tried other approaches through the years, including deep plane facelift, it was my personal observation that an SMAS facelift with 2 vector approach with appropriate submental correction gives the best results. These observations have been documented by others in the literature, including, more recently, the study by Bassichis and Becker in *Archives of Facial Plastic Surgery*. I describe my techniques at the end of the panel discussion.

PERKINS

There are a few advantages to performing facelift techniques that do not require wider subcutaneous skin undermining. The rate of hematoma is not as high with a limited subcutaneous flap like that used in a deep plane classic technique. In addition, the vascular side of the skin flap is a little bit more robust with a shorter skin undermining and a deeper elevation of the SMAS. This may be an advantage in prior smokers. These advantages, however, in my opinion, do not outweigh the benefits of an extended SMAS approach, which takes advantage of not only extended elevation of the SMAS like the deep plane does but also adequate skin undermining for a second vector redraping.

Although the SMAS imbrication technique can dramatically improve the jowl, it provides minimal improvement in the melolabial fold of the midface. Claims of midface-lifting improving this area have not been found to be true. The midface can be defined as the portion of the cheek that encompasses the area between the lower eyelid and the level of the oral commissure.[1] Injectable fillers are advantageous in improving this area. A midfacelift is a procedure that may improve it somewhat but not much.[2]

Extended SMAS facelift with the modified deep plane technique can incorporate dissection just below the zygomatic buttress up over the malar eminence, releasing malar dermal attachments superficial to the zygomaticus muscle and into the midcheek if necessary. Not all patients require elevation of the SMAS in this region. Once good mobilization of the jowl and midcheek tissues has been accomplished with extended SMAS undermining, further dissection into the midcheek may not be necessary. Theoretically, extending the dissection in this region increases the risk of injury to the zygomatic and buccal branches of the facial nerve.

What techniques are most effective in managing the neckline in face-lifting and in what sequence should these be performed?

McCOLLOUGH

As is the case for other areas for which a facelift is indicated, diagnosis precedes treatment. The etiology of an undesirable neckline must be determined. Is it caused by loose skin? Is fat involved? How does the anatomic relationship of the hyoid and thyroid cartilage to the mandible contribute to the cervicomental angle?

If the hyoid bone and thyroid cartilage are titled forward, producing an obtuse cervicomental angle, there is not a lot that can be done (safely) to correct it. If, however, these structures have a vertical orientation, and it is determined that fat is contributing to the problem, fat should be removed with direct excision and/or liposuction. In some cases, it is helpful to remove subplatysmal fat as well.

If the edges of platysmal muscles are divergent (producing platysmal banding), a platysmaplasty (suturing the divergent edges together in the midline) is the most reliable method of correcting the problem. In some cases, a myectomy (removing a V-shaped portion of the muscle perpendicular to the leading edge of the platysmal muscle) may be sufficient. Whenever platysmaplasty is performed, the skin of the neck should be undermined from side to side, connecting the submental wound with the postauricular dissection on each side of the face; otherwise a "cobra deformity" is likely to be noted after swelling subsides.

In virtually all facelifts performed by this author, SMAS suspension in the cheek and posterior neck regions is performed, providing additional improvement in the cervicomental angle. In this author's experience, to obtain optimal improvement of the cervicomental angle, the postauricular incision should be carried posteriorly and inferiorly along the occipital hairline. Experience has shown that when the postauricular incision does not extend to this point, SMAS is not supported to the occipital fascia and the skin is not undermined (as is advocated in some short scar facelifts); as much as 7 cm of skin can be left behind, leading to inadequate treatment of the skin of the neck.

When the neck needs to be addressed at the time of face-lifting, I address it first, performing the procedures mentioned earlier. Then, I perform a cheek/neck-lift with SMAS suspension and skin removal.

The bottom line is that minimally invasive techniques do not provide long-term improvement of the anterior neck, requiring that the surgeon (or a colleague) will often be asked by the patient to perform additional surgery within months after the first surgery.

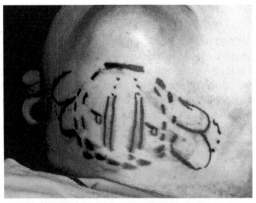

Fig. 5. The patient has areas of attention in the submental area marked in the preoperative room with the patient in the upright animated position.

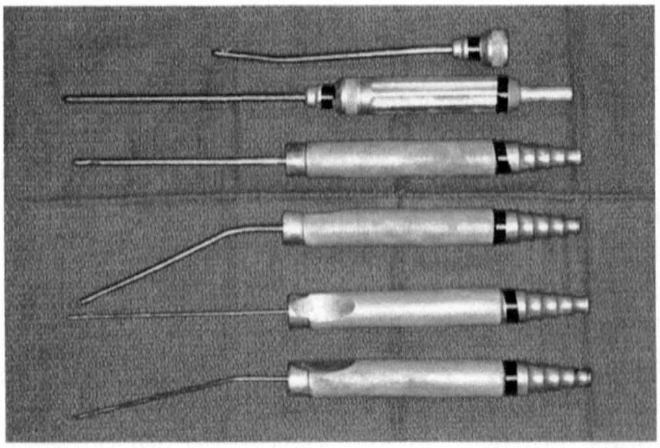

Fig. 6. A variety of liposuction instruments are available, but the author prefers small diameters of 2 to 4 mm in size.

THOMAS

Most patients benefit from a combination of submental liposuction, removing the adipose content of the mandibular line and submental area combined with tightening of the platysmal layer. These are the 2 maneuvers that most frequently contribute to an aesthetic neckline (**Figs. 5–7**).

PERKINS

Surgery to improve the neckline requires operating on the neckline itself. Facelift techniques that do not directly approach the anterior neck often fail to improve the neck in most patients. Platysmal laxity, cervical liposis, and midline submental fat cannot be adequately addressed solely through a preauricular incision of any type. The foundation for a pleasing cervical mental angle is the platysmal "sling" that is created by midline platysmal placation and posterior anchoring of the platysmal/SMAS flap (**Fig. 8**). This is a key element in achieving an excellent and a lasting cervical mental angle and good neckline in face-lifting. Often this is really important for patients who are seeking rejuvenation of their face and neck.

I prefer to perform submental/jowl liposuction and corset platysmaplasty at the beginning of the case for several reasons. This is very important because I have tried to do the platysmal tightening after having posteriorly pulled the platysmal and have had many lateral recurrent platysmal bands occur because of inadequate formation of the corset with subsequent sling. I always elevate the neck skin before making the preauricular incision. With this technique, it is easier to approximate the muscles in the midline before they have been pulled posteriorly. Also, extremely important, I prefer to have a strong platysmal "unit" before advancing the platysmal posteriorly. I use the platysmal portion of the SMAS-platysma flap as a sling and do not excise it. I attach it to the posterior mastoid periosteum, as described in the synopsis of my procedure section.

As noted in the face-lifting article by Patel and Perkins,[2] this sequential cauterization, excision, and suturing of the platysmal and submental fat from the mentum and submental incision, posteriorly to the submental angle, creates a firm anterior corset that sets the stage for bilateral posterior suspension and imbrication of the platysma.[3] Some contouring at the cervical mental angle from the wedge excision of the platysmal and subplatysmal fat in this area only may be required in heavier necks to actually create the angle.

The senior author (S.P.) has found that aggressive techniques in the region of the neck have

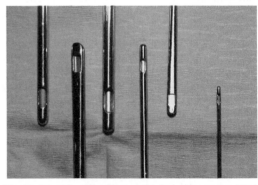

Fig. 7. Cannulas that have a single hole on one side is preferable and the spatula-shaped tip is often helpful.

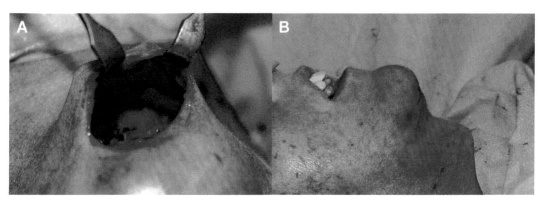

Fig. 8. (*A*) Completed anterior suture imbrication of the anterior borders of the platysma from the submentum down to the cervical mental angle where bilateral "wedges" of platysma have been excised. (*B*) Intraoperative result of a patient after liposuction of the neck and Perkins' Kelly clamp technique for anterior corset platysmaplasty has been completed before posterior sling/suspension.

dramatically improved the overall initial long-term results for the neck portion of the rhytidectomy[2] with thus a much happier patient population overall.

Liposuction of the neck and jowls is an essential part of creating a sharp neckline (**Fig. 9**). Over-zealous liposuctioning can create contour irregularities and an oversculpted look; however, most women have some cervical liposis and fat in the jowl region that cannot be corrected with SMAS and platysmal work alone. When performed correctly, liposuction is an excellent additional technique to improve the results not only of the neckline but also of the jawline in face-lifting.

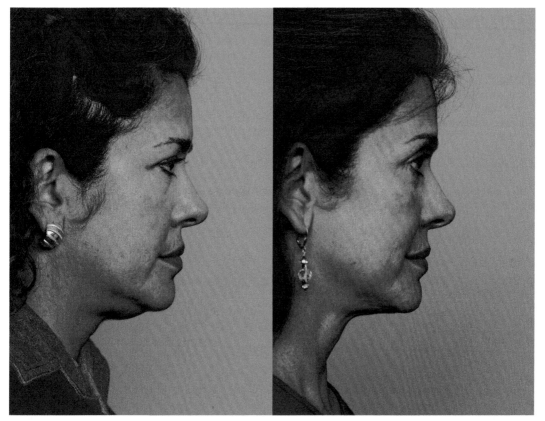

Fig. 9. A 43-year-old woman who underwent liposuction only of the neck, jowl, and jawline, producing a very noticeable result without any platysmaplasty or facelift technique.

Which, if any, face-lifting techniques have been proved to provide the longest lasting result?

McCOLLOUGH

After having performed more than 5000 facelifts, I do believe that some variations of the procedure (particularly those that suspend the deeper tissues in the face and neck with fascia-fascia sutures) enhance both short- and long-term results. Other techniques and principles that are beneficial include the following:

1. Selective low-pressure crisscross liposuction (**Fig. 10**) along the mandibular margins to remove fatty tissue in the jowl region
2. Excisional lipectomy and low-pressure liposuction in the submental region to remove unwanted fat
3. Anterior platysmaplasty in necks with prominent platysmal banding and in necks with an obtuse cervicomental angle (**Fig. 11**)
4. In virtually all facelifts, I excise a strip of fat and fascia overlying the parotid gland (**Fig. 12**), lift the leading edge of the distal edge of the defect, dissect the SMAS free from the underlying tissues (as described in question number 1), and use fascia-to-fascia closure of the resulting defect with multiple (10–12) interrupted 2-0 Vicryl sutures (refer to **Fig. 36** in the Approaches and Techniques section). Placement of each of these suspension sutures is critical. An "accordion" technique is used to gain a purchase of the distal SMAS advancement flap. The proximal purchase of each stitch incorporates the proximal edge of the defect that was created with the initial fat/SMAS excision (refer to **Fig. 36** in the "Approaches and Techniques from the Masters" section). Suture placement is repeated 10 to 12 times, until a semicircular row of interrupted sutures has been created, securing the distal SMAS flap to fascia, including that overlying the occipital muscles, particularly in patients at stages III to V. Except for point-specific contouring purposes, avoid suturing fat to fat, regardless of the suturing technique used. If suspension of facial and neck tissues is the objective, sutures placed in fat are effective but for a short time and eventually pull through, causing the surgical anastomosis to break down and distal tissues to sag more rapidly

5. When planning surgical incisions for face-lifting, make sure that the postauricular incision is extended along the posterior hairline to allow removal of the excess skin from the neck after posterior suspension of the platysma with its enveloping SMAS has been accomplished, especially in patients with class IV and class V conditions. So-called short scar and other minimally invasive proprietary lifts that do not include postauricular and occipital hairline incisions often leave behind from 4 to 7 cm of skin that could have been removed from the neck and, therefore, are destined for disappointment in patients with class III, IV, and V conditions.

THOMAS

In my opinion, the longest lasting result is variable with the technique used and the skill of the surgeon as well as with the physical characteristics of the patient. There is no question that those

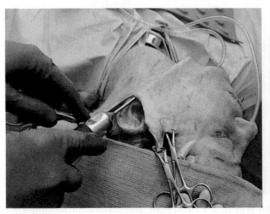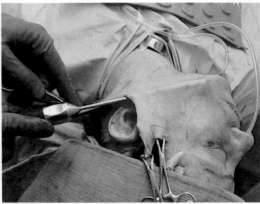

Fig. 10. (*Left* and *right*) Multidirectional low-pressure suction-assisted lipectomy.

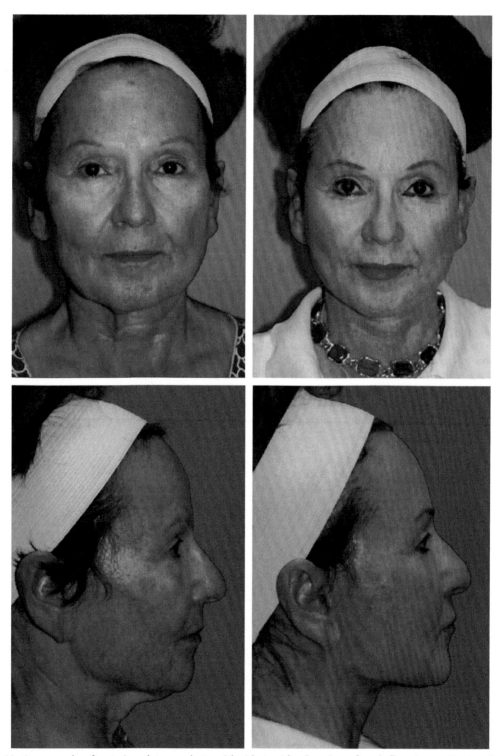

Fig. 11. An example of anterior platysmaplasty with side-to-side elevation of neck flaps in a patient coded as SQ-3, V-2, CH-3, Mar-2, Ne-4, DL-3, FX-2, WR-2.

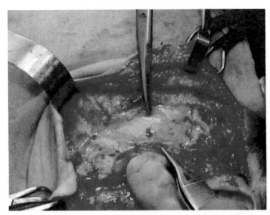
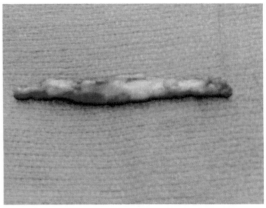

Fig. 12. (*Left*) Excision of fat and SMAS over parotid gland. Note free edges of fascia. (*Right*) Strip of fat and fascia removed.

patients with better muscle tone and skin tone and who tend to be at a somewhat younger age and with less UV exposure tend to do better. Similarly, there is a familial and genetic variation of elastic and collagen fibers of the skin and their ability to respond to the aging process. Finally, of course as noted, it is difficult to compare results from one practitioner to another based on individual skill levels and multiple variations of technique. Nevertheless, it is my opinion, and that of others, that no other technique other than properly done SMAS technique seems to provide a longer lasting result. I describe my face-lifting techniques at the end of the panel discussion.

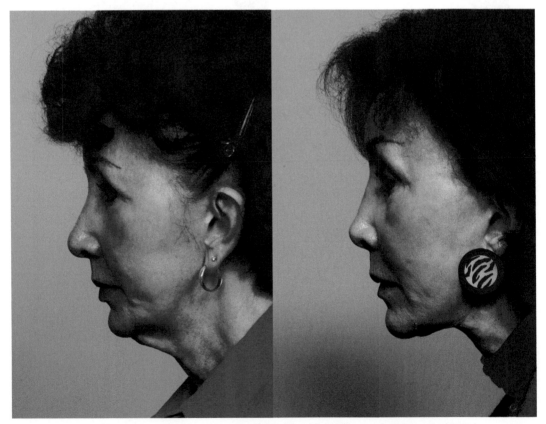

Fig. 13. A 64-year-old woman with a 3-year result of facelift with midline corset platysmaplasty.

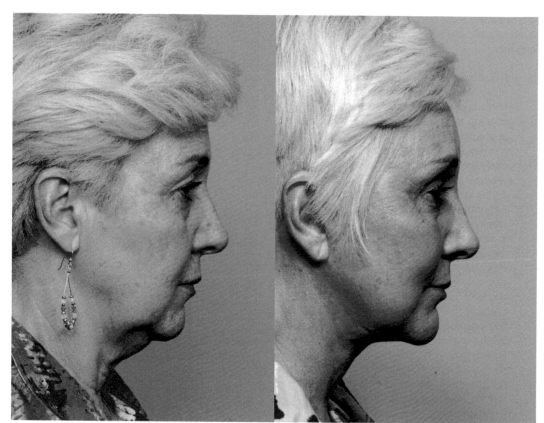

Fig. 14. A 62-year-old woman with full-extended SMAS facelift with platysmaplasty and minimal improvement in melolabial folds 2 years postoperatively.

PERKINS

Performing a midline corset platysmaplasty, as described in the previous discussion, is the foundation for excellent, natural, and long-lasting results in the neck (**Fig. 13**). On the other hand, there is no technique at all that has been proved to provide long-term results in the jowl region or the melolabial folds (**Fig. 14**). Some additional maneuvers to vertically lift the jowl tissues have helped prevent the lateral swoop look that can be a telltale sign of previous facelift surgery. Vertical vectors to the SMAS tissues help to alleviate this problem and also enhance the midface.

To start, develop, and maintain a busy face-lifting practice, is it necessary or even beneficial to offer some sort of minimalist facelift procedure (ie, short scar) or even a noninvasive substitute procedure?

McCOLLOUGH

For a beginning surgeon, the best answer for this question is to exercise good judgment and operate within the scope of his or her training and experience. If a "minimalist" facelift procedure (ie, short scar lift) is the only technique that a surgeon feels qualified to perform, that is the procedure he/she should perform. However (and this advice is as important as any that I can offer), patients should be informed, in advance, by the operating surgeon that the facelift he or she is offering is a minimalist facelift and that the results will not achieve what more invasive procedures can accomplish.

Otherwise the legal burden of informed consent, covering alternatives of treatment, will not have been met.

- Patients should also be told that additional minimalist procedures can be performed from time to time to address recurrent sagging. In some cases, multiple less invasive procedures could be a viable alternative to more extensive surgery, especially in nicotine users and in patients with advanced cardiovascular disease or diabetes.
- Trying to venture beyond one's expertise and perform maximally invasive techniques when one is not experienced in such procedures invites disasters—the kinds of disasters that a growing practice simply cannot afford.
- Promising more than some minimally invasive or nonsurgical techniques can deliver, however, will quickly bring a surgeon's credibility into question and destroy a fledgling practice before it has a chance to get off the ground.
- Nonsurgical procedures can never accomplish what well-advised and well-executed surgery can achieve. Patients must always be told the truth about any treatment; otherwise patients lose confidence in the surgeon and are quick to tell their friends about their own disappointing experiences. Unhappy patients will not fail to provide the name of their surgeon to anyone who will listen.
- The following is the bottom line for the surgeon: investigate the advantages and disadvantages of each and every technique, device, or material that one intends to incor-

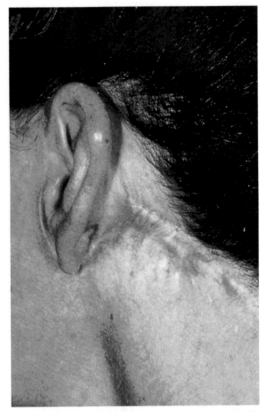

Fig. 15. A postauricular widened scar created by the surgeon closing with too much tension.

porate into his or her practice and make sure that it can achieve the claims made by those promoting it; then, operate within one's limitations and refer when indicated.

THOMAS

Regardless of whether the surgeon is developing a new practice or maintaining an ongoing established practice, the key is to have good results with a happy patient population. To suggest that some minimalist procedures are a good way to start and then move on into more involved procedures simply fails to recognize that the procedure should be selected to best correct the individual patient problems. Importantly, in an aesthetic elective procedure such as facelift, it is essential to pursue a procedure that not only gives good results but also minimizes the risk of complication (**Figs. 15–20**). Noninvasive treatments such as fillers, Botox, or other resurfacing procedures certainly can be important adjuncts to the facelift procedure. However, so-called liquid facelifts and other similar marketing-orientated descriptors may be misleading to patients and should instead be thought of as treatments for those individuals who do not require surgical intervention or as adjuncts to facelift.

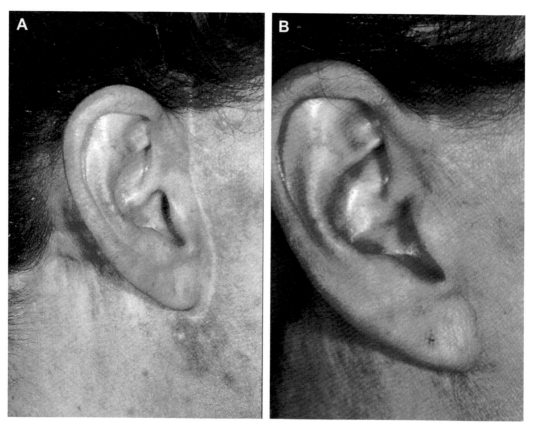

Fig. 16. (A) Inappropriate placement of the incisional scar by the original surgeon. (B) The patient after excision of the scar and advancement of skin to create a posttragal incision line and a scar position better camouflaged at the cheek/ear junction.

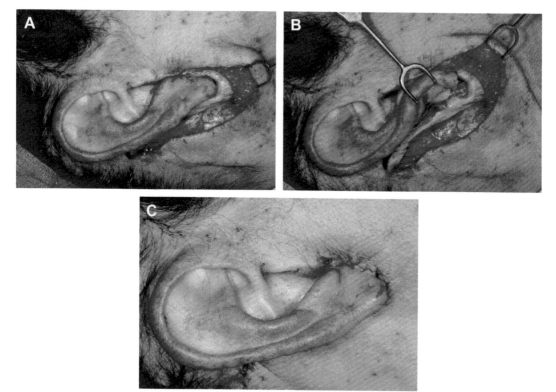

Fig. 17. (A) Correction of the auricular scar begins with reincision distal to the scar. (B) The scar and intervening skin is excised. (C) The skin flap is advanced and closed in proper position.

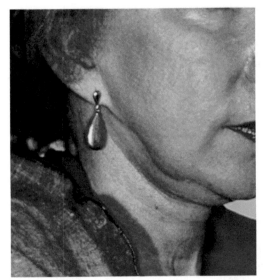

Fig. 18. The "pixie" ear deformity following the surgeons closure with too much skin tension in the infra-auricular region.

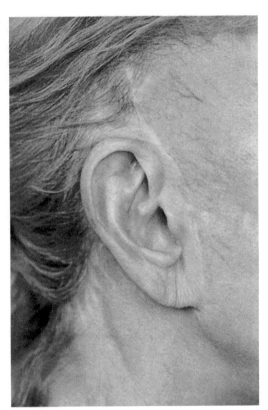

Fig. 20. An example of the surgeon advancing and overcorrecting the temporal area, creating hairline deformity.

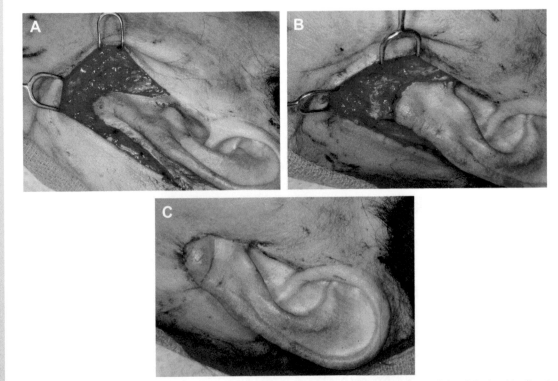

Fig. 19. (*A*) Correction of the "pixie" deformity begins with incision adjacent to the earlobe. (*B*) The skin flap is elevated, and the scarred earlobe is sharply released from underlying scar. (*C*) The flap is elevated to create an earlobe cleft, and the lobe is repaired.

PERKINS

Providing a lesser operation for patients who need facelift is detrimental to developing a successful face-lifting practice. The goal of any cosmetic procedure is to provide pleasing, long-lasting, and natural results, resulting in happy satisfied patients. Patients who need a facelift deserve a complete operation, not a minimalist operation that either fails to provide the result they desire or has very short-term benefits. Compromising with a short scar procedure may be an attractive marketing tool, but it leads to suboptimal results and dissatisfied patients (**Fig. 21**). This is an antithesis to building a reputation as a good facelift surgeon in one's community. Doing the proper operation, resulting in happy patients who refer other patients to their surgeon because of the good results achieved, not only in the face but also in the neckline, and having scars that are minimally noticeable, is a stronger marketing tool than any other technique that can be used to attract patients. In fact, trying to short cut the facelift operation results in either a minimal improvement or so much tension on the skin that there are widened, visible scars and pulled-down earlobes, giving the patient cosmetic deformities that are not only telltale signs of having had a facelift but also need to be corrected or camouflaged. These patients will seek care elsewhere or refer their friends elsewhere. If their friends see those kinds of scars or results, they may choose not to have a facelift at all.

Similarly, I do not believe there is any noninvasive substitute for patients who actually need a facelift. There are modalities that heat the tissues, which creates some temporary tightening of the deep dermal layer and subcutaneous tissues. These often need to be repeated and are usually performed with expensive lasers using infrared wavelength techniques. Radiofrequency heat is similarly bulk heating and creates temporary effects with a fair amount of pain. There are some ultrasonic techniques and machines available to create true subcutaneous wounding, and current modalities are being tested to actually

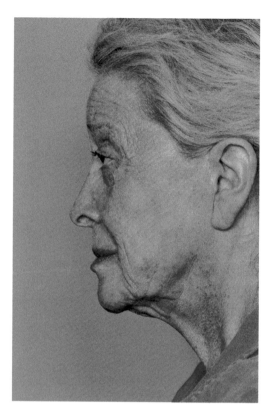

Fig. 21. A woman in her late 60s who underwent a short-incision facelift and received a very minimal result in the cheek and no result in the neckline. In addition, she now has visible scars that cannot be camouflaged by makeup or hairstyle.

heat the subdermis in a fractionated manner. These show some promise for at least some visible results that may last 1 to 2 years (**Fig. 22**) for patients who are waiting to have a facelift or who are, at this point, not ready to commit to having a standard facelift operation; but there is no substitute to a well-done facelift with a good foundation because it serves the patient well for many, many years. Unfortunately, there are patients, young and old, who have undergone Ulthera treatment and have either no result or minimal visible results (**Fig. 23**).

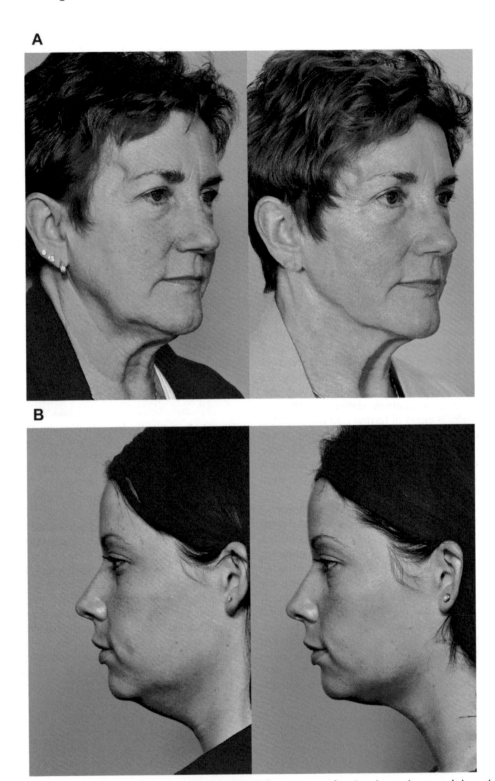

Fig. 22. (*A*) A woman in her late 50s who underwent high-frequency profractional sound wave subdermal treatment to the cheek and jawline and was happy with the minimal results. (*B*) A woman in her late 20s with neck and jawline lipoptosis who had a noticeable improvement from Ulthera (high-frequency–focused sound wave energy delivered in a linear manner in subcutaneous and subdermal tissues).

A

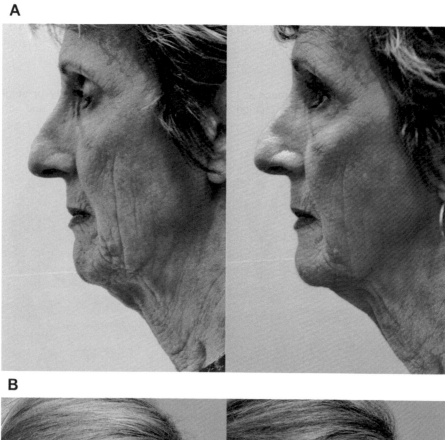

B

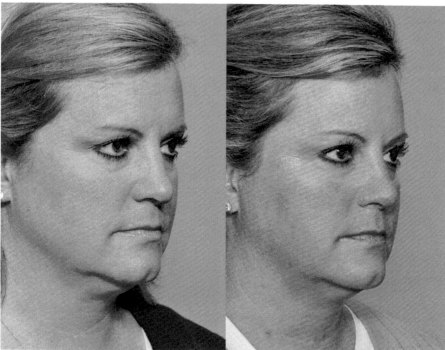

Fig. 23. (*A*) A woman in her late 50s with significant loss of elasticity who insisted on a noninvasive technique and refused to have a standard facelift. She underwent Ulthera treatment with minimal results. (*B*) A woman in her early 40s with jowl and neck lipoptosis who underwent 2 Ulthera treatments and received no appreciative results.

Analysis: Over the past 5 years, how has your technique or approach changed or what is the most important thing you have learned in performing facelifts?

McCOLLOUGH

I still perform the facelift operation very much as I have over the past 30 years. The major change would be that, in the stage IV or stage V neck with large amounts of fat and an obtuse

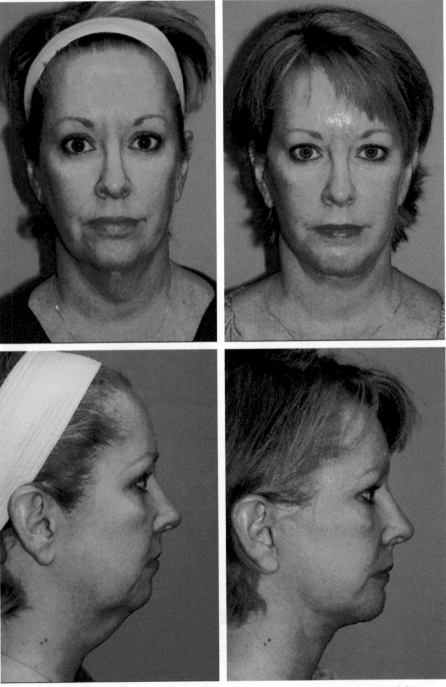

Fig. 24. Example of neck-lift, incorporating suction-assisted lipectomy, anterior platysmaplasty, and chin augmentation.

cervicomental angle, I have found that anterior pla-tysmaplasty (suturing the leading borders of the muscles together, along with midline subplatysmal fat excision) and side-to-side undermining of the skin flaps provide a better result (**Fig. 24**).

I also continue to be superimpressed by tricho-phytic face-lifting incisions, made in a beveled fashion a millimeter or so behind the hairline in the forehead, sideburn, and postauricular region. When incisions are made in this manner, hairlines are preserved and, when the technique is per-formed properly, hair grows through the scars to provide camouflage (**Figs. 25** and **26**).

From my own teachers and mentors, I learned that it pays to rely on techniques that comply with the basic principles of surgery—truisms learned by every physician while attending medical school. In my own practice, I affirmed many of those same tenets.

The following list of ruminations is offered in hopes that they may be of benefit to my colleagues and the patients for whom they care:

1. One of the greatest obstacles for patients contemplating facial rejuvenation to over-come is the fear of looking "pulled" or "stretched." If a surgeon can demonstrate that he or she only performs surgery and ancil-lary procedures designed to produce a natural appearance, patients are much more likely to go forward with treatment.
2. The only reliable closure of deep tissue defects is one that approximates fascia to fascia, and multiple interrupted sutures are more reliable than a single continuous suture.
3. The most reliable method of avoiding perma-nent injury to a nerve, blood vessel, or anatomic structure is to refrain from dissect-ing or cauterizing close to it.
4. The aging process is a continuum and varies from patient to patient. The best facelift can be improved upon at a future date by mainte-nance procedures that are designed to address many of the same conditions treated at the time of the initial surgery.
5. The length of time between an initial facelift and the need for a "tuck" or maintenance procedure are not always under a surgeon's control. Factors that speed the aging process and cause tissues to prematurely sag include emotional stress, poor nutrition, genetics-based life expectancy, illness (either in the patient or in someone close to the patient), or the death of a loved one.
6. Better is the enemy of "good." Every opera-tion, and every nonsurgical treatment, follows the gaussian bell-shaped curve. There is a point of maximum benefit, beyond which risks outweigh benefits.
7. New is not necessarily better. It takes 5 to 7 years before any new technique or modifica-tion of an existing technique can be said to be better than the one currently in use.
8. In evaluating candidates for facial rejuvena-tion, chronologic age is irrelevant. It is the bio-logical age of the skin, face, and neck that matters most.
9. No practice-building scheme has ever come close to the time-honored one based on word of mouth. Satisfied patients tell their friends and family about a good experience and a natural-looking result. They are also quick to share unpleasant experiences with everyone they meet.

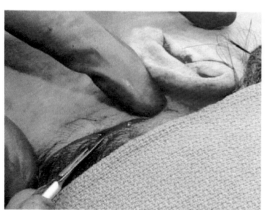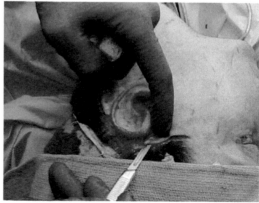

Fig. 25. (*Left*) Postauricular and occipital beveled trichophytic incision. (*Right*) Temporal sideburn beveled tricho-phytic incision.

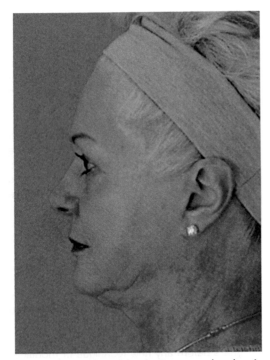

Fig. 26. Patient after trichophytic temporal and occipital incisions. Note hair growing through and below the scars.

10. Being honest with patients is the best way to earn, and maintain, their trust and respect.

11. Being honest with one's self and working within the limitations of one's training and experience minimizes the likelihood of disastrous outcomes.

12. Referring a difficult case to a colleague who has more experience (or expertise) in handling such conditions will help build the referring doctor's own practice much more rapidly than turning out substandard results.

13. Respect for the teachings of great minds and giving credit where credit is due earn a physician the respect and admiration of his/her colleagues.

14. Initiate change with skepticism. Only fools believe everything they hear—or read. Check out the claims of too-good-to-be-true schemes, products, or techniques and investigate the reputation of the people making them.

15. Incorporate the "lagniappe" or "baker's dozen" philosophy in your practice. Whenever possible offer something extra...at no extra charge. Deliver more than patients bargain for.

16. When uncertainty raises its head, the way forward lies within the Golden Rule.

THOMAS

The technique I have described has evolved over the past 30 years of practice. Over that period, I have tried several other alternative approaches, including deep plane facelift. However, the procedure described here and that I refer to my trainees as the safety facelift has given me overall consistently happy patients and avoided complications. I describe my techniques at the end of the panel discussion.

PERKINS

Over the past 5 years, I have made several subtle modifications to my facelift approach. I have been less aggressive with submental liposuction and more aggressive with midline platysmaplasty. The reason I became a little less aggressive with submental liposuction is because I had created a few dermal bands at the cervical mental angle. A layer of fat needs to be left on the skin, both subcutaneously as well as deeply, to avoid creating dermal bands that are difficult to eradicate. In addition, submandibular liposuction, if overdone, can actually create visible submandibular glands, which, in my opinion, should not be excised. One has to accept the fact that, occasionally, a more ptotic submandibular gland becomes more visible after face-lifting but should not overaggressively perform liposuction and create the problem, if possible. I continue to be extremely pleased with the midline platysmaplasty in creating a neckline that lasts. There is still a 1% to 2% submentoplasty tuck-up rate in my practice on an annual basis taking all patients as a collective group. This is an acceptable submental reoperation rate that is dramatically less than it was before the corset platysmaplasty that I now perform.

I have significantly increased the use of prejowl implants in patients with heavy jowls and/or deep preoperative prejowl sulci (**Fig. 27**). This has been a wonderful addition to face-lifting not only in the initial contour and visible appearance but

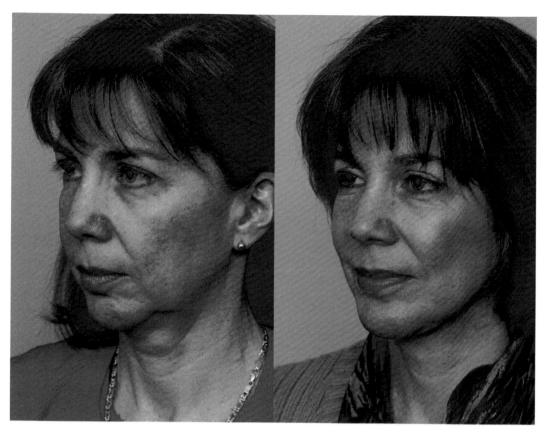

Fig. 27. A woman in her early 50s who desired improvement in her jowls and neckline and presented with a hypoplastic mentum and deep prejowl sulcus. She successfully underwent a standard SMAS rhytidectomy with Mersilene mesh chin implant and a Silastic Mittelman[10] prejowl implant.

also in the prevention of or early recurrence of the jowling appearance in patients who are bound to have settling in this region. Patients tolerate this extremely well, and I have had no complications with prejowl implants. Chin augmentation is performed as necessary but as a separate augmentation of the mandible issue.

I have greatly increased the use of hyaluronic acid fillers in the nasolabial folds and marionette folds at the time of surgery. I even use some calcium hydroxyapatite in weak chin-cheek regions to bolster this area because it is not improved with a standard facelift procedure. Downward turn of the oral commissure of the mouth is not improved without some filling or improvement of this groove directly.

I no longer perform temporal incisions (see previous discussion). I did this many years trying to achieve smoothing in the temporal region and obtained a minimal effect in lifting the lateral brow. I was constantly trying to make sure I did

not raise an already high hairline and made several modifications in the inferior sideburn region. I finally gave up using temporal incision entirely. If a temporal lift is required, it is a separate incision that is performed as a separate operation. The cheek portion of the facelift does not require any temporal extension. In this sense, my scar has shortened dramatically and the amount of dissection in the temporal region is essentially none.

I have also increased the number of combined midfacelifts with facelifts (**Fig. 28**); however, I do not perform midfacelifts on greater than 10% of my facelift population because the vertical pull of the SMAS adequately treats the midface in most patients.

Fortunately, the fundamental technique I use for performing facelifts has not changed over the last 15 to 20 years. It has provided excellent natural long-term results with happy patients, the ultimate measure of success for any surgeon. Videos showing technique for facelift are available online:

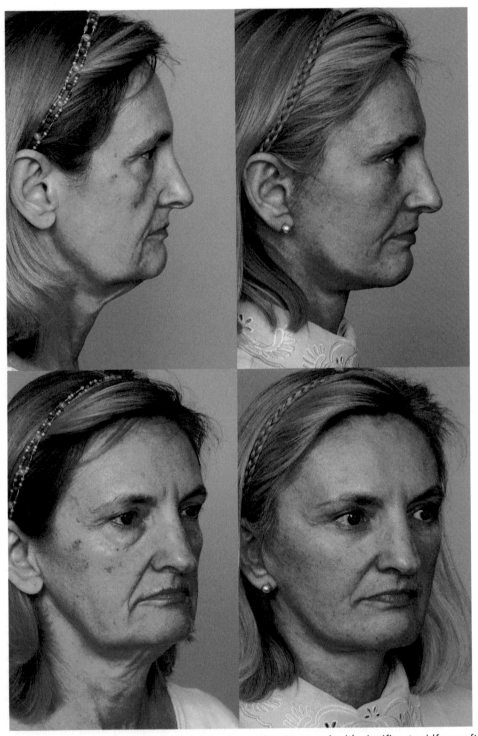

Fig. 28. A woman in her early 60s desiring facial rejuvenation presented with significant midface soft tissue atrophy and descent and successfully underwent a standard SMAS rhytidectomy in addition to a midfacelift.

FACELIFT APPROACHES AND TECHNIQUES FROM THE MASTERS

McCollough: A Synopsis of My Approach to Facelift, Addressing Controversies

For generations, facial plastic surgeons, including I, searched for the ideal facelift. In the early part of the twenty-first century, however, it occurred to me that there is a reason why the holy grail of facial rejuvenation has not been discovered. We surgeons have been looking in all the wrong places. We have been quick to follow colleagues promoting procedures, and practices, that ignore the time-honored canons of surgery. Cleverly titled one-size-fits-all-faces techniques have only added further confusion. A growing number of doctors are joining commercial ventures that offer too-good-to-be-true solutions to an unsuspecting public.

Realizing that there was a need to redirect the profession's focus back toward reason, I set out on a mission to develop a condition-specific classification system and algorithm that could be used for facial rejuvenation. Initially, I began to use the system in my own practice. Then, my thoughts and experience were offered to colleagues during presentations at scientific meetings. In 2010, my work was published in the peer-reviewed medical literature (**Figs. 29** and **30**).

The system I created is based on measurable parameters that help determine the biological age of each anatomic region of the face and neck. By doing so, I am able to create a condition-specific treatment plan and rely on that plan to recommend, and perform, the right combination of procedures for each patient, regardless of the patient's chronologic age.

For example, a younger (stage I-A) face (**Fig. 31**) might only require suction-assisted lipectomy along the lower jawline and neck. A cheek or temporal lift (with or without liposuction) might be indicated in patients in stage 2-A (**Fig. 32**), whereas in a stage IV face, a forehead, temporal, cheek, and neck-lift with or without liposuction and platysmaplasty and a subsequent skin resurfacing procedure might be indicated (**Fig. 33**). No one-size-fits-all face-lifting technique can provide this kind of versatility, even if the term *extended* is added to its title. Also, so-called short scar procedures leave behind several centimeters of skin in the neck (**Fig. 34**). Although a vertical vector cheek-lift tightens sagging neck tissues in the short run, the effect is short lived. It is, therefore, my conclusion that the most reliable method of addressing the neck (with a facelift) is to extend the incision behind the ear and along the occipital hairline.

Like skin incisions, the extent of skin undermining varies from stage to stage and is determined

---

"Face lift" is the term commonly used to describe a surgical procedure better known in medical circles as "rhytidectomy" (removal of loose, wrinkled skin of the face and neck). The procedure is designed to re-create the firmer, smoother face of youth. However, not all *face lifts* are the same – nor should they be! The reason is: *not all faces are the same.* And, at different ages the same face is a different face.

Dr. McCollough's system is comprised of five (5) general treatment plans:

STAGE I (The Less Than Thirty Face Lift): for the younger individual who has little or no loose skin and may require only liposuction to remove unwanted fat and bulges.

STAGE II (The Thirty-Something Face Lift): for the patient who is beginning to notice sagging of the brows and cheeks, *but not the neck*. Whenever sagging tissues are present, facial muscles and fat must be repositioned into their more youthful relationships. In such cases a small amount of loose skin is removed.

STAGE III (The Forty-Something Face Lift): for the patient who exhibits sagging brows, cheeks and neck. Some of these patients may or may not need liposuction for contouring jowls and fullness under the chin. All, however require suspension techniques to muscles and fat .

STAGE IV (The Fifty-Something Face Lift): for the patient with *generalized* facial and neck sagging, with – or without – jowls and wrinkles around the mouth. With more obvious muscle, fat, and skin laxity, more suspension of these structures is required.

STAGE V (The Sixty-Plus Face Lift): for the patient with *advanced* aging, coupled with sagging of all facial areas, including the forehead, brows, cheeks, and neck. At this stage in the aging process, deep folds develop in the groove between the nose and face, jowls droop below the jaw line, and the muscles of the neck often produce string-like bands that run vertically from the chin to the upper chest. Many of these patients are also beginning to exhibit wrinkles and blemishes over most of the face

Fig. 29. The McCollough Face-Lifting Classification System.

MCCOLLOUGH CONDITION-SPECIFIC FACIAL REJUVENATION CLASSIFICATION

PATIENT'S NAME: _____ RECORD NUMBER: _____ DOB: _____ ☐ MALE ☐ FEMALE

EVALUATOR: _____ ☐ ATTENDING ☐ FELLOW ☐ OTHER _____

☐ INITIAL CONSULT ☐ FOLLOW-UP DATE OF EVALUATION _____

PREVIOUS PROCEDURES: _____

FACE LIFT CLASSIFICATION

STAGES	ASA	PSY	FH	T	CH	NE	PL	ML	MAR	EAR R	EAR L	up-1/3	mid-1/3	low-1/3 Buc	low-1/3 Lip-up	low-1/3 Lip-low
0																
I																
II																
III																
IV																
V																
SURGEON'S RECOMMENDATION																
PATIENT'S DECISION																

FACELIFT ANNOTATIONS:
ASA: American Society of Anesthesiologist Physical Status
PSY: Psychological Readiness
FH: Forehead
T: Temporal
CH: Cheek
NE: Neck
PL: Platysmal Banding
ML: Melo-labial Groove
MAR: Marionette Groove
EAR: Earlobe
V: Volume
R/L: Right/Left
V: Soft Tissue Volume
up: Upper
mid: Middle
low: Lower
1/3: Da Vinci's Horizontal Thirds
Buc: Buccal Fat Pad
Lip-up: Upper Lip
Lip-low: Lower Lip

UPPER EYELIDS (UEL)

STAGES	FX R mfp	FX R nfp	FX L nfp	FX L mfp	SX R	SX L
0						
I						
II						
III						
IV						
V						
SURGEON'S REC						
PATIENT'S DECISION						

LOWER EYELIDS (LEL)

STAGES	FX R ofp	FX R mfp	FX R nfp	FX L nfp	FX L mfp	FX L ofp	SX R	SX L
0								
I								
II								
III								
IV								
V								
SURGEON'S REC								
PATIENT'S DECISION								

EYELID ANNOTATIONS:
FX: Fat Excess
SX: Skin Excess
ofp: Orbital/Lateral Fat Pod
mfp: Middle Fat Pod
nfp: Nasal Fat Pod

RESURFACING ANNOTATIONS:
GSS: Global Skin Score (the mean of all SQ & WR scores)
UPORB: Upper Peri-Orbital
LPORB: Lower Peri-Orbital
UPORL: Upper Peri-Oral
LPORL: Lower Peri-Oral
NOS: Nose
GLA: Glabella

SKIN RESURFACING CLASSIFICATION

STAGES	GSS	SQ (SKIN QUALITY) FH	T	CH	UPORB	LPORB	UPORL	LPORL	NOS	WR (WRINKLES/RHYTIDES) FH	T	CH	UPORB	LPORB	UPORL	LPORL	GLA
0																	
I																	
II																	
III																	
IV																	
V																	
SURGEON'S REC																	
PATIENT'S DECISION																	

DATE OF SURGERY: _____ SURGEON: _____

Fig. 30. The McCollough Condition-Specific Facial Rejuvenation Classification.

by the degree of biological aging in each anatomic region (see **Fig. 29**). Except in stage I-A lifts, SMAS suspension is performed. If the SMAS is to be a part of a lifting procedure, it is important to free it from its underlying tissue attachments far enough anteriorly and inferiorly to allow mobilization and suspension of the muscles of the cheek and neck. Anatomically, sub-SMAS elevation should be carried just anterior to the parotid gland (**Fig. 35**). I can see no logic behind dissecting far enough into the cheek to expose branches of the facial nerve, especially for surgeons who do not already have a vast amount of experience in performing the facelift operation.

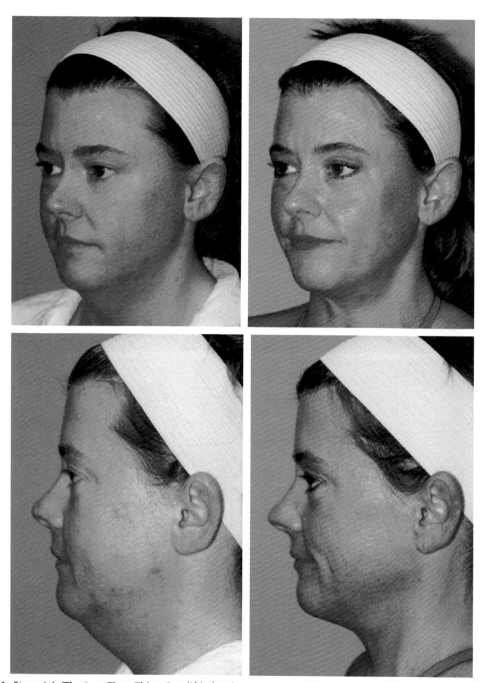

Fig. 31. Stage I-A (The Less Than Thirty Facelift): for the younger individual who has little or no loose skin and may require only liposuction to remove unwanted fat and bulges. Before and after suction assisted lipectomy of cheeks and neck.

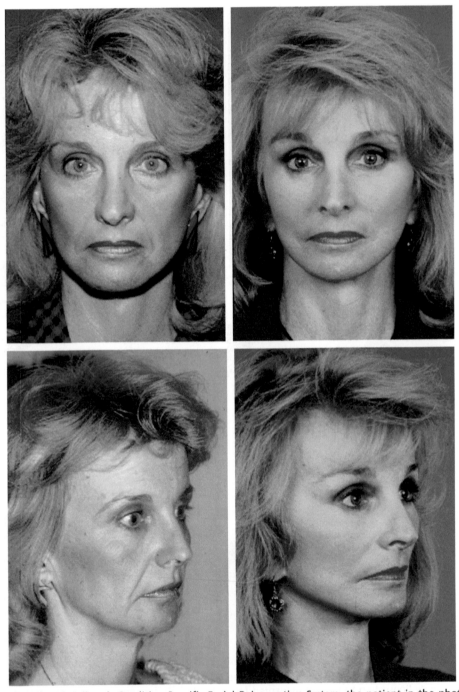

Fig. 32. Using the McCollough Condition-Specific Facial Rejuvenation System, the patient in the photographs would be coded as SQ-2, V-1, FH-2, CH-2, Mar-2, Ne-1, PL-1, FX-2, WR-1. This patient underwent a temporal cheek-lift with SMAS suspension. No eyelid surgery or resurfacing was performed.

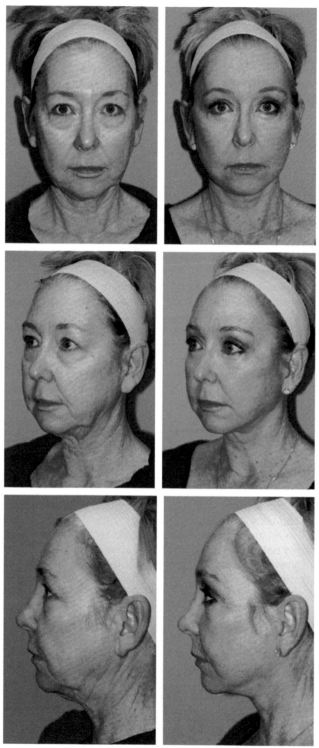

Fig. 33. Stage IV patient who underwent temporal cheek and neck-lift with suction-assisted lipectomy of cheeks and neck and upper and lower eyelid blepharoplasty. Coding score was SQ-3, V-3, CH-4, Mar-3, Ne-4, PL-2, FX-3, WR-3.

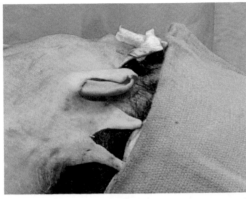
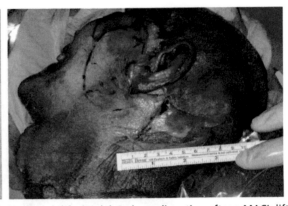

Fig. 34. (*Left*) Patient undergoing stage IV temporal cheek neck-lift. (*Right*) Cadaver dissection after a MAC's lift had been performed. Extension of postauricular incision with SMAS suspension in the neck allowed for 7 additional centimeters of skin removal.

I make every attempt to see that the SMAS advancement flap is anchored, proximally, to fascia that has been denuded of its overlying fat. I do not adhere to the school of thought that fat-to-fat plication results in the kind of favorable healing that suspends the tissues of the face and neck for an appreciable length of time.

Multiple (8–10) interrupted, absorbable sutures (with a half-life of at least 6–8 weeks) are used for SMAS suspension (**Figs. 36** and **37**). Within 6 weeks, a sheet of favorable scarring (that becomes incorporated with SMAS-fascia) should provide the strength needed to support the tissues of the face and neck.

Thomas: Personal Approach to Facelift

Like all facial plastic surgery procedures, there are a variety of approaches and techniques available to the surgeon. Selection of these techniques and approaches are related both to the surgeon's preference and experience and to the specific goals and requirements of the patient. Although my approach to any specific patient is tailored to

Postoperatively, compression dressings are used over undermined areas. I am not an advocate of drains and/or tissues sealants. All dressings are removed the morning after surgery. Detailed printed instructions for aftercare are given to patients and their caregivers.

In short, the McCollough Condition-Specific Classification System is rooted in fundamental surgical principles and uses an algorithmic approach to address the conditions at hand. In time, I predict that such a condition-specific system will supplant one-size-fits-all facelift methodologies and allow surgeons to select and perform the right combination of procedures for the right patient, at the right time in a patient's life.

the anatomic needs and the aesthetic goals of that patient, I typically use a 2-vector SMAS facelift technique that uses specific steps to avoid possible complications while achieving an acceptable result. Because of these 2-fold goals, I often refer to this approach as the safety facelift when discussing this with fellow surgical colleagues

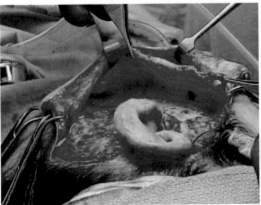
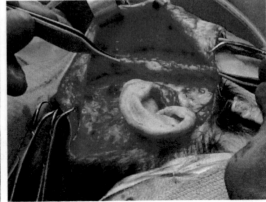

Fig. 35. (*Left*) SMAS flap elevation. (*Right*) Advancement of SMAS flap.

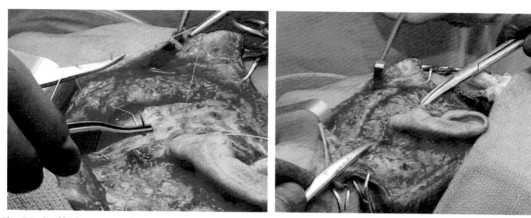

Fig. 36. (*Left*) Placement of SMAS suspension suture. (*Right*) Anastomosis of facial edges after placement of ten 2-0 Vicryl interrupted sutures.

and trainees. This technique uses, as noted, an SMAS level facelift where each basic step of the facelift technique has been examined, the alternatives for each of those steps explored, and an alternative is selected that provides appropriate results while creating comparatively less risk for possible complication. This is done for each step of the facelift as identified in the overall operation and results in the procedure as described.[4]

The anatomy and physiology of facial aging is well understood and documented. The clinical changes observed are further influenced by genetic background as well as by environmental influences, including UV exposure and smoking. These anatomic changes and predictable variables create what is seen in terms of clinical appearance in the aging face. There are, of course, variables with each patient based on those noted factors as well as the patient's age during evaluation and while providing surgical recommendations.[5] There are several procedures described for facelift, and each of these procedures has strong proponents who have a variety of perceptions as to what serves the patient best. Through

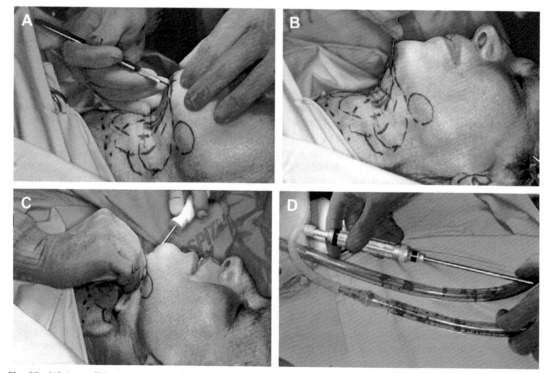

Fig. 37. (*A*) A small incision is initially made in the submental line to initiate liposuction. (*B*) The precise subcutaneous plane is initially created with small scissors. (*C*) Liposuction is performed with a to-and-fro action of the cannula with gentle manipulation of the cutaneous tissue with the surgeon's opposite hand. (*D*) Often significant adipose tissue is removed through this technique.

the years, my personal approach has evolved around the 2-vector SMAS facelift, with attention to specific steps in regard to safety as described here. This approach may be altered in certain situations, including the relatively young patient with early changes that would benefit from a less invasive procedure with smaller incisions or the patient in whom a secondary facelift needs to be performed who eventually requires a touch-up revision after initial procedure previously. This technique evolved after experiences with a variety of other techniques and a realistic evaluation of the results. This personal experience has been reinforced by the observations of others, including several reported in the literature.[6,7]

What these observations all demonstrate in similar fashion is that the ultimate results from an SMAS facelift were comparable to the results of a deep plane facelift technique. Likewise, evaluation of various surgical steps involved would also argue that an SMAS-type technique has less morbidity and less risk of complication. Again, the ultimate goal for a facelift procedure should be an appropriate level of improvement along with minimum risk to the patient for complication in this elective aesthetic procedure.[8]

Steps in Facelift: Thomas

The basic steps of facelift have been established as:

1. Incision planning
2. Submental correction
3. Flap elevation
4. SMAS elevation
5. Closure.

For each of these key steps, various differing techniques have been evaluated, and the one with the least potential risk for complication while accomplishing appropriate improvement has been selected. The first of these is incision planning.

Incision Planning for Facelift: Thomas

In addition to developing access to the tissues, the placement of incisions should avoid visibility of the scars and is of key importance to the patient. Although, as is true for each step, incision planning is based to some degree on physician preference. The one typically selected by this author's experience is to adapt the most inconspicuous and yet utilitarian incision for the individual.

- In the temple area, it is important to hide the incision while giving access to the upper portion of the facelift procedure.
- Attention should be given to avoiding shifting of the hairline as well as making the incision less visible.
- It is preferable to avoid a pretrichael incision because of the potential visibility. Although pretrichael incisions have the potential advantage of avoiding the shift of the hair tuft and temporal hair-bearing area, the visibility of the scar is always potentially present.
- A curvilinear incision starting above the ear and behind the hairline in the temporal region has proved to be superior in most situations. This hides the incisional scar within the hair-bearing skin. A curvilinear incision rather than a straight vertical incision helps interrupt the forces of contracture while avoiding significant shift of the hairline. This incision typically begins 2 to 4 cm above the superior helix and is designed in a C-shaped manner.
- The preauricular portion of the incision is typically a posttragal incision to further hide the scar, which then curves around the auricular lobule and tucks tightly up into the earlobe cleft of that region.
- If the patient has an earlobe anatomic configuration that does not have an inferior earlobe cleft, it is created for the patient to further hide the scar.
- The incision then follows an area on the postauricular concha above the sulcus by 3 to 5 mm. This incision tends to shift postoperatively to fall precisely within the postauricular sulcus and thus hide the incision.
- The incision continues in the postauricular area to the point that would correspond to the superior portion of the external auditory canal and then crosses the sulcus to go into the posterior hairline.
- A small dart or "V" configuration is made over the sulcus to allow for the tissue to fall within that depression and avoid any contracted bridging scar. This incision falls into the posterior occipital hairline and is positioned in a curvilinear manner with attention to positioning the incision so it falls parallel to the hair follicles and thus encourages hair growth postoperatively.

Submental Correction: Thomas

Following decisions on incision placement, typically the first step addresses the submental area. This includes removing adipose tissue through liposuction and, in most patients, plicating the submental platysmal bands and often excising some small amount of submental redundant skin.[9]

- Patients with poor chin projection may benefit from an augmentation chin implant, which may be done through this same incision to further enhance individual appearance and help create a cervical angle.

- Liposuction is accomplished using a small liposuction cannula through the submental incision and done in a radial manner. This is extended into the jowl area to further enhance the jawline. Typically, the initial liposuction is done through a small incision smaller than 1 cm to help maintain negative pressure.

- Following completion of the liposuction, the incision is enlarged and a submental flap in the subcutaneous plane is elevated. This exposes the platysma musculature. The medial margins or bands of the platysma, if redundant, can be excised.

- A subplatysmal flap is then created to allow for advancement and plication of the platysmal muscles in the midline, which is done with a 4.0 absorbable suture.

- A key step is the development of the cervical angle. The platysma is divided at the desired level of the cervical angle, and the margins of the divided muscle are cauterized in a horizontal manner for 1.5 to 2 cm on either side. This division of platysma is often referred to as breaking up the verticality of the platysmal bands. At this point, the flap can be advanced, and usually a small amount of redundant or excess skin is excised before closure.

- Closure is done in 2 layers with a 5.0 absorbable suture in the dermis and 6.0 polypropylene sutures for closure.

- Hemostasis has been maintained throughout this procedure with bipolar cautery, and typically there is no drain used.

Flap Elevation and SMAS Correction: Thomas

- Using the incision designed as described, the facelift flap is then elevated. The flap is elevated in the subcutaneous plane and extended out into the midface area with what has been described as an intermediate flap (Fig. 38).

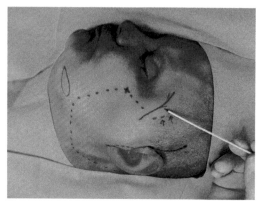

Fig. 38. The typical degree of intermediate flap undermining is indicated on this cadaver specimen. Note that the path of the frontal branch of the seventh nerve is indicated and is carefully avoided with flap elevation.

- This degree of flap elevation contrasts with a short flap that elevates a few centimeters in the preauricular and periauricular area. It likewise is elevated to a lesser extent than a long flap that may extend medially toward the midline of the face into and beyond the nasolabial folds and perhaps connect submentally to the opposite side.

The concept of intermediate flap is that it allows excellent exposure to SMAS layer, allows appropriately draped skin, yet avoids the dissection in the region in which the facial nerve would be more superficial and at greater risk for injury. It also has the effect of minimizing the amount of potential dead space postoperatively and thus decreases the likelihood of hematoma. This again is an operative step in which multiple alternatives to flap elevation are present. This particular approach allows for appropriate surgical correction, while at the same time minimizing the exposure of possible complications.

- This flap extends to the level of the maximal projection of the maxilla and is essentially midway in the face between the auricle and the nasolabial fold.
- The underlining continues inferiorly past the mandible to the neck inferiorly below the inferior portion of auricle and extends postauricularly into the occipital hairline.
- Hemostasis is maintained throughout the procedure with bipolar cautery.
- It is important to stay below the level of the hair follicles in the occipital and temporal areas.
- In the temporal area, the preferable level is deep to the hair follicles and superficial to the temporal fascia and within the loose plane over that fascia.
- Elevation and spreading with scissors often accomplishes most of this elevation in this region.

SMAS Elevation: Thomas

With elevation of the flap, the SMAS is now exposed and available for treatment (**Fig. 39**).

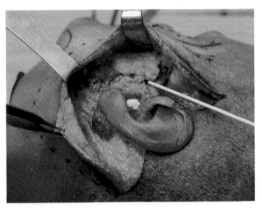

Fig. 39. Following elevation of the skin flap in the subcutaneous plane, the SMAS is evident. The position of the SMAS incision is indicated on this specimen.

- Typically the SMAS layer is elevated with scissor-spreading dissection. Judgment is made as to how much redundant SMAS is available and the dissection is not advanced beyond that point. Once again this ensures the safety of the deeper structures (**Fig. 40**).

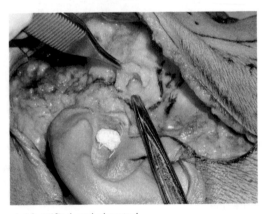

Fig. 40. A distinct SMAS layer is identified and elevated.

- The redundant or excess SMAS is excised, and the remaining SMAS is advanced and tightened, typically in 2 directions or vectors. Thus the 2-vector approach gives appropriate elevation of the SMAS and improves facial support.

- Typically the SMAS in the preauricular area is elevated superiorly, whereas the lower vector beneath the ear and cervical area is projected more posteriorly.

- The SMAS flap is secured in this area with interrupted buried 3.0 absorbable sutures.

- Once the SMAS has been secured, the skin flap is redraped. This allows for tension at the SMAS area and avoids tension in the skin flap. That tension, should it occur in the skin flap rather than in the SMAS, may create tension lines that are unsightly and nonaesthetic. Tension on the skin closure may potentially lead to a widened or lesser appropriate scar (**Fig. 41**).

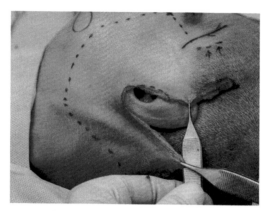

Fig. 41. Following SMAS elevation and plication, the redundant skin is excised with edge-to-edge apposition minimizing tension on the wound. Note the 2 vectors of correction, with the preauricular skin being corrected in a posterior direction vector and the postauricular skin closed in a superior directional vector.

- The skin at this point is excised with edge-to-edge apposition and closed in 2 layers using interrupted 5.0 absorbable sutures in the dermis layer.

- Skin closure in the preauricular areas is with the running subcuticular 5.0 polypropylene suture.

- The posttragal portion is typically closed with a running 6.0 fast-absorbing gut and the postauricular portion closed with 5.0 fast-absorbing gut suture.

- Hair-bearing areas of the temporal and occipital regions are closed with small stainless steel staples (**Fig. 42**).

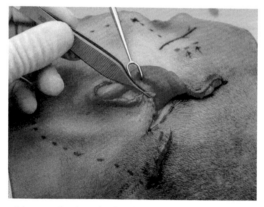

Fig. 42. Careful attention is paid to realigning the hairlines without creating a step-off deformity.

- Because of the precise hemostasis with bipolar cautery throughout the procedure and because of the intermediate flap elevation and the smaller potential for hematoma, routinely a drain is not required.

- At completion of the procedure, the incisional areas are cleaned, antibiotic ointment is applied to all regions, and a nonadherent gauze strip is then applied to the incisions.

- This is followed by a gauze wrap and an elastic dressing for the final layer.

- The dressing is changed the following morning and the patient inspected for hematoma.

- If all is appropriate on inspection, a similar dressing is reapplied for another 24 hours.

- Following removal the next day, the patient is given an elastic chin support to use throughout the remaining week.

- Sutures are removed at 1 week.

Stephen W Perkins, with Assisting Authors Jaspreet K Prischmann and Jonahtan Y Tinj:
A Synopsis of My Approach to Facelift, Addressing Controversies

Following is a synopsis of my approach and controversies I think exist related to my approach versus other facelift techniques and other surgeons' philosophies.

The term facelift has some connotations that are perceived by many patients as negative. A facelift is a standard rhytidectomy procedure that involves improving the neck and jawline and somewhat the midfacial tissues. Many patients desiring improvement in their aging characteristics are particularly bothered by the changes they see in their neck. Therefore, many of them present for consultation requesting a neck-lift and "not a facelift." Although I do agree that the main focus of a facelift is improving the neck and jawline, it inherently involves improving the jowl and cheek tissues simultaneously with adequate and excellent improvement in the neckline. Conversely, improving only the cheek tissues does not necessarily equate with a good facelift procedure because the neckline can often be neglected depending on the technique, and the results will be less than satisfactory.

Therefore, a facelift is, in my opinion, to a greater extent, all about the neck and less about the cheek and jowls. There are exceptions to this in the sense that many patients do have jowling or heavy jowling and cheek tissues as their primary concern, with the neck being a secondary issue for them. Patients must be educated as to what

a facelift is and what a neck-lift is and must be able to determine that they are often a combined procedure. They also must be educated as to what a facelift will do and what it will not do. A facelift is a procedure that is imperfect by its nature yet treats certain underlying aging anatomic issues that exist with almost every patient presenting for midface to lower face rejuvenation.

If the patient is primarily interested in improving his/her smile creases or cheek-lip grooves, then a facelift may not even be the operation for them. There may be other alternatives of treatment that are much more beneficial and more directly productive in terms of improving the issue that concerns them.

There are also patients who have such anatomic heaviness to the midcheek and jowl tissues that a facelift is, at best, a mediocre answer to resolving what bothers them. In fact, they may well need to accept that their preexisting anatomic condition is not significantly improved by any known and proven present-day surgical techniques that we have available to choose from.

It is, however, critically important to diagnose and effectively treat whatever conditions exist in the submental, submandibular, and lower neck to achieve a truly long-lasting and satisfactory result in face-lifting. Improving the cheek and jawline may in fact require more structural surgical

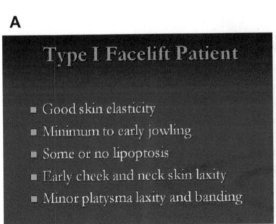
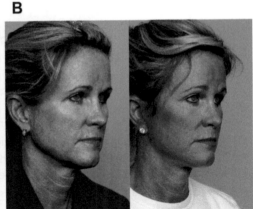

A

Type I Facelift Patient

- Good skin elasticity
- Minimum to early jowling
- Some or no lipoptosis
- Early cheek and neck skin laxity
- Minor platysma laxity and banding

B

Fig. 43. (*A, B*) Characteristics and example of a type I facelift patient.

A

B

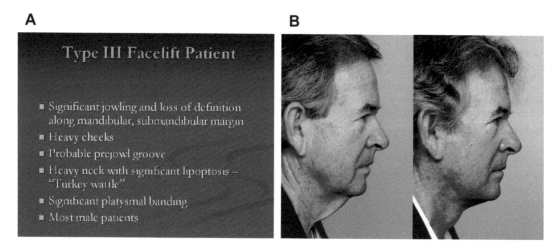

Type II Facelift Patient

- Average type of preoperative patient
- Moderate degree of ptosis of skin, fat and platysma
- Moderate lipoptosis
- Noticeable jowling
- Heavier neck with platysma banding and loss of cervico-mental angle

Fig. 44. (*A, B*) Characteristics and example of a type II facelift patient.

approaches, such as chin augmentation, prejowl implant,[10] and fillers to the midface rather than the standard or a choice of a variety of known facelift techniques.

Therefore, it is important to understand and educate each patient that a facelift is inherently an operation that has definitively known benefits and some lasting results but is doomed to some degree of failure in every case from the short or long term, depending on the patient's preexisting anatomy, heredity and elasticity, social interactions, and overall health condition.

Having said that, facelift is also a very gratifying procedure that helps improve the quality of life for many patients, no matter what their preexisting anatomic, hereditary, or aging condition is. It is my opinion that a facelift operation begins with how to most effectively manage the neck and, secondarily, how one can improve and enhance the jawline, jowling, and midfacial tissues. Therefore, I classify the type and fee for the facelift based on the degree and extent of work required in the neck to achieve an excellent and long-lasting neckline (**Figs. 43–45**).

A

B

Type III Facelift Patient

- Significant jowling and loss of definition along mandibular, submandibular margin
- Heavy cheeks
- Probable prejowl groove
- Heavy neck with significant lipoptosis – "Turkey wattle"
- Significant platysmal banding
- Most male patients

Fig. 45. (*A, B*) Characteristics and example of a type III facelift patient.

Technique: Perkins

It is my philosophy and standard modus operandi in face-lifting to treat the neck first. The neck is treated at the start of the operation to set the stage for maximum improvement of the neckline before any kind of posterior elevation and SMAS suspension is performed. This is somewhat controversial in that there are physicians who believe that posterior elevation and suspension is indicated before any kind of anterior platysma treatment. I personally have approached the operation initially with that sequence and have been more than often frustrated or disappointed in the recurrence of midline and/or lateral platysmal bands based on having not approximated the anterior platysma before posterior suspension.

Liposuction: Perkins

A 2.5- to 3-cm incision is made in the submental crease, depending on the anatomy of the patient, and the skin is elevated for 5 to 10 mm in the subcutaneous layer to allow the introduction of a small, 3-mm, round liposuction cannula. It has become somewhat controversial as to whether or not liposuction is indicated at all in treatment of the neck, but I believe it is crucial to the maximum improvement I can achieve for any given individual patient. I perform some degree of liposuction in more than 97% to 98% of all my facelift patients. A 3-mm round cannula is used with 3 holes lined up on one side to remove fat in a minimalist manner, yet I do move to a larger 5-mm and 7-mm cannula, if required, depending on the amount of fat and the density of tissue in the submental region.

See Video: Submental and jowl liposuction in rhytidectomy.

- Initially, I pretunnel the skin over the jowl overlying the mandibular margin all the way in a radial manner from the anterior border of the sternocleidomastoid down past the cervical mental angle to the other jowl region without any suction applied (**Fig. 46**).

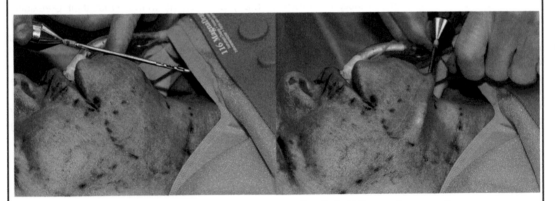

Fig. 46. Pretunneling the neck and jowl with a 3-mm round 3-"holed" liposuction cannula.

- Once I have pretunneled with the 3-mm cannula, I use a regular liposuction machine that creates 1 atm of negative pressure to remove the excess and redundant fatty tissue.
- The lipoptosis that exists, in the jaw, submandibular, submental and full neck areas, is grasped with my nondominant hand and fed into the cannula as I rotate the cannula 270° to the left and to the right.
- Judicious liposuction is used in the jaw area, but I still believe that it is important to defat this area to get the maximum improvement and the long-term longevity to the facelift. Care is taken not to overdo removal of fat, so as not to get dimpling.
- Similarly, despite aggressive liposuction in the submental area, which is required with even a large cannula, is imperative not to injure the dermis or cross the cervical mental angle with any aggressive liposuction so as not to create dermal banding in the postoperative period.
- Injury to the marginal mandibular nerve is avoided on a routine basis by picking up the soft tissue and skin, platysma, and fat and pulling it away from the mandibular margin before introducing the liposuction cannula and performing liposuction.
- Care is taken to avoid overzealous suctioning in the submandibular area to skeletonize the submandibular gland and make it more visible.[11]

Submental Platysmaplasty: Perkins' Kelly Technique

To adequately treat the neck and be able to predictably create excellent long-lasting necklines, I prefer the Perkins' Kelly clamp technique for submental platysmaplasty with every facelift. See Video: Sequential submental excision and plication of subplatysmal fat and platysma: Kelly clamp platysmaplasty.[1] I perform this before any posterior SMAS-platysmal elevation and posterior superior suspension. There are differences in opinion as to whether the platysmaplasty should be performed before the posterior pull of the platysma and superior posterior pull of the SMAS. In my opinion, the platysmaplasty technique sets the stage for the ability to create a natural sling of the patient's own soft tissues to suspend the neck and create the sharpened neckline. See Video: Submentalplasty in rhytidectomy: Wide skin undermining and Kelly clamp platysmaplasty. If one were to perform the platysmaplasty after the posterior pull, it occasionally prevents the ability to plicate and imbricate the platysma in the midline and one loses the effective and natural sling suspension. In addition, when inevitable relaxation occurs, the laterally displaced anterior borders of the platysma become lateral platysmal bands and give the illusion of a "cobra" deformity.

- I favor the use of a 5-in curved Kelly clamp for the submental platysmaplasty because it provides safe reliable results without prepredicting the amount of platysma to be excised.

- Complete undermining of the neck skin with a Kahn beveled facelift dissection scissors is required to separate the skin from the platysma and perform the platysmaplasty through the submental incision. See Video: Undermining post auricular neck skin flap in rhytidectomy.

- The elevation is carried across the cervical mental angle and the anterior border of the sternocleidomastoid bilaterally.

- The loose anterior platysmal bands and the redundant midline subplatysmal fat are then cross-clamped with this large curved Kelly clamp in the anterior midline.

- Then, starting from the level of the incision in the submentum, sequential cauterization, direct excision with Metzenbaum scissors, and immediate buried suture imbrication of the platysmal borders is accomplished with 3-0 Vicryl sutures (Ethicon, Somerville, NJ, USA) (Fig. 47). One can do this in an interrupted manner or by using figure-of-eight sutures. Occasionally this is supplemented by 2 buried 3-0 Tevdek sutures that are permanent in nature if the patient has a neck that is very heavy or particularly adipose.

Plication versus imbrication is a matter of definition. There is really no foldover of the platysma. It is an end-to-end approximation of the predetermined excision, which is grasped between the Kelly clamp at the beginning of the procedure. The sequential excision suturing is done from the submental crease down to the cervical mental angle.

See Video: SMAS imbrication: undermining, advancement, and suturing of the SMAS/platysma as a sling suspension in rhytidectomy.

- A wedge of platysma and fatty tissue is excised at the angle on either side of the imbrication laterally. This takes care of any platysma bands that are extending down more inferiorly in the neck and allows a sharp angle to be created.

- Occasionally, subplatysmal fat in this region is excised and this is the only area where subplatysmal fat is directly excised that is not within the clamp initially. A firm anterior corset is thus created, setting the stage for bilateral posterior suspension and imbrication of the platysma.[3]

- The neck skin is undermined completely to redrape these tissues in a posterosuperior manner, and the neck skin is moved in a different vector.

- Inferior sideburn and preauricular and postauricular incisions are then created, first on the right side of the face and then on the left. It is imperative that one takes care to maintain the preauricular tuft of hair following the preauricular curvature of the helix from its superior insertion to its root inferiorly.

- Incision is not carried into the temporal hairline tuft. It either is at the inferior aspect of the sideburn tuft of hair or creates a new inferior aspect of the sideburn tuft at the level of insertion of the helical/anterior helical rim.

- Incision is then carried posttragally in all female patients and even some male patients. Incision then continues around the earlobe. The postauricular incision rises slightly above the sulcus in the medial aspect of the auricle to allow for postoperative settling of the scar in the postauricular sulcus.

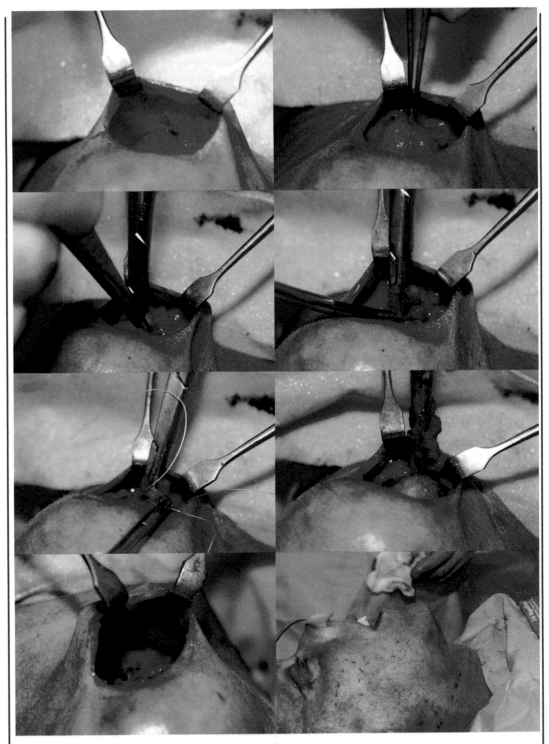

Fig. 47. Perkins' Kelly clamp corset platysmaplasty technique.

- At the level of the eminence of the concha postauricularly, the incision is curved gently toward the hairline at about the level of where the helical rim touches the posterior hairline. It crosses the non-hair-bearing portion very high, so the resultant scar is not visible.

- It extends either horizontally and then inferiorly into the occipital scalp for patients with minimum to moderate skin laxity (**Figs. 48** and **49**) or occasionally will be brought down and along the postauricular hairline before the tail of the incision is brought back into the occipital scalp. This is done for patients with greater skin laxity and redundancy in the neck.[12] It is much more common that I prefer placing the incision into the posterior occipital scalp so as to hide it completely, and the patient can wear their hair in any style, a ponytail, or otherwise on top of their head.

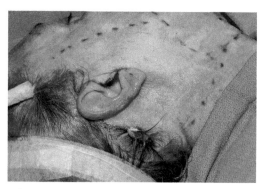

Fig. 48. My preferred outline of preauricular and postauricular incisions for a typical facelift patient.

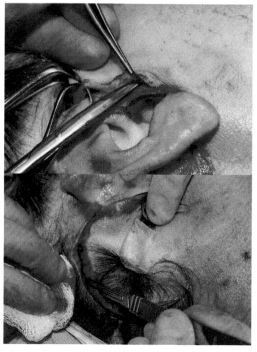

Fig. 49. Making the preauricular and postauricular incisions for a face-lift.

Skin Flap and SMAS Elevation

Attention is then turned to skin flap elevation.

- Using a blunted Kahn beveled facelift scissors with the tips up in an advancing, spreading technique, the skin flap can be elevated, ensuring the dissection is in the proper plane, a plane that leaves fat under the surface of the skin flap but on top of the SMAS and platysma (**Fig. 50**).

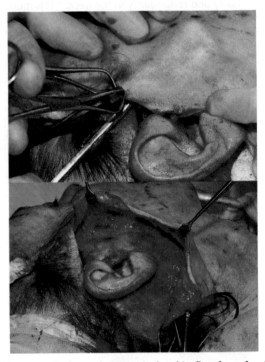

Fig. 50. Scissor elevation of the preauricular and postauricular skin flap for a facelift.

- A postauricular skin flap is first elevated in a plane deep to the hair follicles and superficial to the fascia of the sternocleidomastoid muscle and then immediately more superficial into the immediate subcutaneous plane. This is to ensure that the elevation does not pass deep to the fascia or the sternocleidomastoid muscle, which could then allow injury to the greater auricular nerve. By staying superficial to the fascia, the greater auricular nerve is preserved. This dissection is a bit more difficult because of the attenuation of the fat in this area and the stronger dermal attachments of the skin to the fascia.
- Once past this region, dissection is carried easily into the subcutaneous intra-adipose plane, moving the elevated neck skin flaps from the submental incision elevation.
- Elevation of these skin flaps allows visualization down inferiorly beyond the mandibular margin of the neck. The skin flaps are elevated between 4 and 6 cm preauricularly and again continuously from ear to ear across the neck.
- Separating the skin flap from the platysma is imperative because the suspension, anterior imbrication, corset platysmaplasty, and posterior sling suspension are performed as a separate layer vector than the redraping of the skin. No bunching or dimpling occurs.
- The skin flap is left in continuity with the SMAS in the midface and anterior face so as to allow elevation of the midfacial tissues and jowl when the SMAS is suspended.[12]
- Once hemostasis is obtained, the incision is made starting at the inferior border of the zygomatic arch at the level of the lateral malar prominence. It is extended diagonally from this position to the bottom of the earlobe and continues inferiorly 1 cm in front of the anterior border of the sternocleidomastoid (**Fig. 51**).

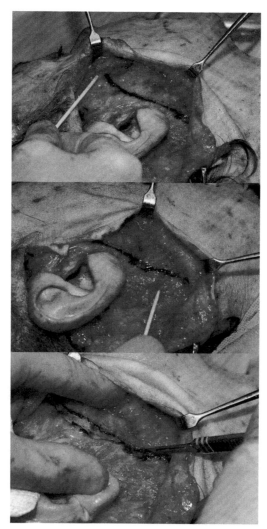

Fig. 51. The incision through the SMAS and posterior platysmal in the preauricular region and anterior to the sternocleidomastoid muscle.

- Once the incision is made in the SMAS, dissection is performed with a Metzenbaum scissors in a first horizontal spreading manner, separating the SMAS and platysma from the superficial layer of the deep investing fascia of the parotid gland. Dissection is carried up to 3 to 4 cm beneath the platysmal muscle. The marginal mandibular nerve can be visualized occasionally but is below the fascia investing the masseter muscle.

Attention is then turned to the midcheek region and elevation of the SMAS of the cheek.

- Dissection begins just below the zygomatic-malar maxillary buttress in the sub-SMAS plane, extending to the inferior aspect of the orbicularis muscle. This dissection frequently requires release of strong dermal attachments to the malar eminence, and the dissection is extended superficial to the zygomaticus major muscle and further into the midcheek if necessary.

- Not all patients require full SMAS elevation of the midcheek, as has been reported with a standard defined deep plane facelift.[13] I elevate the SMAS in this region just far enough to allow mobilization of the SMAS 3 to 4 cm superiorly and posteriorly, gaining good cheek elevation.

- Once good dissection inferior to the malar area is in a separate deeper plane, deep to the zygomaticus muscle but inferior and superficial to the zygomatic and buccal branches of the facial nerve, I extend the dissection on top of the masseter muscle just far enough to get good sufficient mobilization of the jowl tissues. This modification of the deep plane technique increases safety by decreasing the risk of injury to the zygomatic and buccal branches of the nerve, as they are under direct visualization.

It is an extended SMAS elevation imbrication technique combined with a separate skin flap elevation with partial deep plane connections to the skin flap as one extends past 4 to 6 cm in the preauricular region.

Suspension of Midface and Jowl: Perkins

At this stage, suspension of the midface and jowl tissues is accomplished by advancing the SMAS in a superior and slightly posterior manner. The superior vector to the SMAS is critical while elevating the jowl and even submental deeper tissues. There is partial elevation of the platysmal muscle in this vector, but the strong elevation is of the cheek tissues. Some posterior movement is also obtained in the preauricular area.

- *The SMAS is not excised.* The superior slip or a significant portion of the SMAS is left intact and suspended to the dense preauricular tissues near the periosteum of the posterior aspect of the zygoma. This is about the level of the helical insertion, and a 0 Vicryl suture is used for the strength of this firm suspension. Tremendous movement in the jowl or midcheek tissues occurs with this one suspension suture.

- At the level of the earlobe and just slightly superior to this, a cut is made into the SMAS-platysma flap, and it is split. The inferior aspect of the flap, which is primarily platysma and some SMAS, is then suspended in a more posterior and somewhat superior manner.

- *The platysmal flap is not excised!* See **Fig. 52.** A 0 Vicryl suture is used to suspend this platysmal flap, sliding over the sternocleidomastoid and fascia to the periosteum of the mastoid. This sharpens the neckline tremendously because the now natural corset sling platysmaplasty is completed.

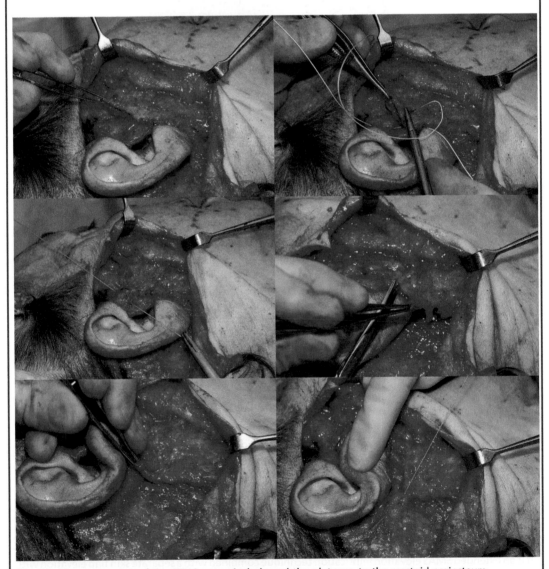

Fig. 52. Sling suspension of the SMAS preauricularly and the platysma to the mastoid periosteum.

- There is occasionally some redundant fat and the posterior border of the platysma flap that is trimmed extending more inferiorly into the neck. The redundant portion of the SMAS in the preauricular region, which is about 2 to 3 cm long and 1.5 to 2.0 cm redundant, is trimmed with the Metzenbaum scissors.

- The SMAS in this region is imbricated end to end with 3-0 monocryl dissolvable sutures (3-0 polydioxyl suture; Ethicon, Somerville, NJ, USA), as is the posterior edge of the platysma flap, as it is draped over and sutured to the posterior fascia investing the sternocleidomastoid muscle.

- The skin flap is easily advanced superior and posteriorly up and on the auricle and in a more posterior vector, the check, leaving only about 2 to 3 cm of undermined skin in the preauricular region.

- The skin of the neck is advanced more superiorly and slightly posteriorly, taking great care to align the posterior hairline so as not to get a step-off deformity (Fig. 53).

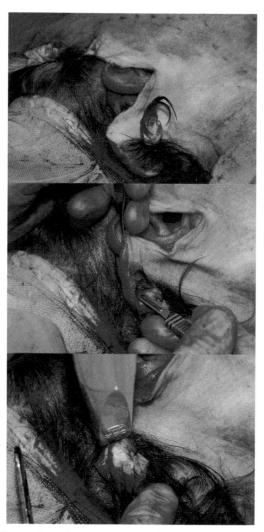

Fig. 53. Advancing the skin flap and aligning the postauricular hairline.

- These 3 different vectors are achieved in an effect similar to that described by Baker with a triplane rhytidectomy.[14]

- The hair-bearing portions of the scalp, just at the inferior aspect of the sideburn and postauricularly from the posterior hairline back into the occipital scalp, are closed with staples.

- The skin is closed with a few buried 5-0 monocryl sutures and running interlocking 5-0 plain catgut suture.

- Two 6-0 nylon sutures are placed at the bottom of the earlobe and left in for 10 days to assure good healing of the earlobe because it swells and is under some upward tension to prevent a satyr ear deformity or pixie ear.
- The preauricular skin is moved into a more posterior and superior vector to avoid any undue movement in the temporal tuft or sideburn hair and not chasing a dog-ear anteriorly.
- Redundant preauricular skin is trimmed, creating a tragal flap that is redundant and sutured under no tension in a running interlocking manner with 5-0 plain catgut suture. There is some thinning of this flap if there is fat underlying this, so as not to make the tragus too fat. The tragus will then not be pulled forward, and the patient will have no preauricular scar as a telltale sign of the facelift.
- Before closing the earlobe portion of the wound and the postauricular portion of the wound with 5-0 plain catgut suture, a 7-mm ribbed drain is placed and brought out the postauricular scalp and placed on each side of the lower anterior neck, about 6 cm.
- It is then connected to a closed suction bulb drainage (**Fig. 54**). This has reduced rates of seromas and hematomas significantly in my practice compared with not using drains.[15] This also allows a light compression dressing consisting of an ABD or abdominal dressing combined with a light Kerlix wrap.

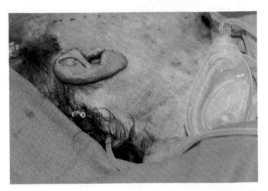

Fig. 54. A 7-mm ribbed drain in place in the neck connected to closed system bulb suction before application of light compression dressing.

- A nonstick dressing is placed around the ear with antibiotic ointment before placement of the mild compression dressing. There is no pressure on the skin flaps whatsoever so as to avoid venous congestion, which increases the possibilities of infection and skin flap failure.
- All sutures and staples, except the earlobe sutures, are out and removed at 7 days.

CONTROVERSIES AND COMPLICATIONS IN FACELIFT

Stephen Perkins Addresses Additional Controversies and Complications Related to Extended SMAS Rhytidectomy

The art and science of face-lifting involves performing enough surgery to create the desired results. Each procedure is tailored to the individual patient's preexisting anatomy, inherent elasticity, and desired and needed improvement. There is no one facelift procedure that fits all, but some standard tenants do apply. Proven, safe, reliable techniques supersede all other modifications to the facelift procedure. Proponents of limited, minimally invasive, or short scar operations generate, in my opinion, limited; minimal; short-term; or, in some cases, untoward negative results.

Controversy 1: Does Elevating the Subcutaneous Flap Create Contour Irregularities?

Wide undermining of a subcutaneous flap creates some temporary contour irregularities during the immediate postoperative period. Most of the time, undermining just a bit further, smoothing out any dimpling or irregularity at the time of the surgery, prevents many of these. Fortunately, any irregularities that do exist in the immediate postoperative period usually dissipate within the first 1 to 3 weeks. Small persistent irregularities can be treated with in-office intralesional steroid injections. They are hardly ever permanent. Proponents of deep plane and short scar face-lifting are often made to manage unsightly "bunching" in the preauricular and postauricular regions, respectively. In my estimation, this is much less of an initial aesthetic outcome than redraping the skin and tailoring it appropriately and adjusting the length of the skin incision based on the elasticity and needs of the patient.

Controversy 2: Does an Extended SMAS Rhytidectomy Have Enough Vertical Pull?

My technique for rhytidectomy allows for advancement in multiple vectors. The preauricular SMAS flap is advanced significantly superiorly and then superolaterally. It incorporates the vertical pull of other so-called vertical facelifts, such as the MACS lift. The postauricular SMAS flap is advanced posterolaterally, a great deal posteriorly, and some superiorly. Similarly, but in a different plane, the preauricular skin is advanced, tension free, mostly laterally and slightly superiorly.

The postauricular skin is advanced somewhat posteriorly and superolaterally and a bit anteriorly. This multiple-vector technique creates consistently natural, lasting results and maintains hairline continuity in all cases.

Controversy 3: Should Subcutaneous Undermining Continue to the Melolabial Fold? Are There Any Techniques That Improve This Area?

I do not perform undermining subcutaneously to the melolabial fold. Such wide undermining can create an unnatural, "pulled skin" look that is difficult to correct or that may never relax. This gives face-lifting a "bad name," leaving people looking unnatural and as though they are too taut or as if standing in front of a fan. Despite some believing that a deep plane facelift improves the melolabial fold, I am unaware of any short- and long-term studies that have corroborated this claim. This region can only be improved with adjunctive procedures, that is, midfacelift to some degree, mostly fillers, and occasionally direct excision of the fold.

Controversy 4: Is it Necessary to Extend the Facelift Incision into the Hairline Posteriorly? Is a Temporal Extension Necessary Anteriorly?

It is absolutely necessary to extend the facelift incision into the posterior hairline. In my opinion, at least extending the incision across to the hairline and down the postauricular hairline before tucking the end into the hairline is required to redrape the skin and take as much neck skin redundancy away as possible. There is no other way to redrape the neck skin without creating bunching or "dog-ears." Folds in the postauricular area take a long time to settle down, and there is minimum ability to remove skin when stopping the incision high in the postauricular sulcus and not extending it posteriorly. Advocates of short scar procedures must deal with redundant postauricular skin. Where does this skin really go? It does not go anywhere and is not really removed.

Extending the incision into the hairline requires precise realignment of the postauricular hairline at the time of closure. It does not generate additional complications or downtime. On the contrary, it prevents unsightly postauricular bunching, and an incision in the postauricular scalp is not an issue. The only issue is the scar that goes down to the nape of the neck, and, even if one follows the postauricular hairline for most postauricular scars, it still needs to be posteriorly directed into the scalp so that it is not visible with any hairstyle in which the hair can be brought posteriorly, as in a ponytail or with the hair up on the head. A well-designed scar brought up as high as the helical rim, touching the postauricular hairline, and then posteriorly into the scalp allows women to wear any hairstyle they so choose.

I rarely perform a temporal incision. It not only raises the hairline but also takes additional time and dissection. I have not found it to be useful in lifting the temporal region, or lateral brow, to any great extent. It certainly adds nothing specifically to the facelift if the proper skin redraping is performed. If one pulls too vertically on the cheek flap, one will have folds in the temporal region that have to be addressed. The answer to this is to not raise the skin in that vertical direction and not create the folds.

Controversy 5: Are Dressings or Drains Necessary After Facelift? Are Fibrin Sealants Advantageous?

Over the past 28 years, I have tried numerous postoperative regimens. My current regimen, which is one I have used most of the nearly 30 years I have been performing facelift, involves a light kerlix dressing and, in the past 20 years, includes the use of drains. I have found that very light pressure dressings are helpful not only for hemostasis but also for camouflaging and cushioning the surgical field. I have tried to avoid drains but have consistently found anywhere from 4 mL to 6 mL of drainage collecting in the first 12 hours at some place under undermined skin flap. This is particularly true with the degree of undermining I believe is required in the neck skin to create a bi-planar vector to maximize the neck results. The skin is separated from the platysmal muscle completely. The use of drains has minimized the creation of hematomas and seromas to approximately 3% to 4% of patients, and the use of a light compression dressing has minimized any kind of venous congestion or endangerment of the viability of the flap. Tight compression dressings have a significant risk of creating some areas of focal necrosis.

Fibrin sealants, of which I have tried every brand several times, in my hands, have resulted in an unacceptable incidence of seromas. About 85% to 90% of facelifts in which I used fibrin sealants resulted in at least small, if not multiple, seromas. I no longer use fibrin sealants. One other issue with fibrin sealants is the cost involved in using the sealants in a private practice setting. There is a cost associated with drains, but it is about one-fifth the cost of fibrin sealants at this time.

SUPPLEMENTARY DATA

Supplementary data related to this article can be found online at http://dx.doi.org/10.1016/j.fsc.2012.02.001.

SUGGESTED READINGS: McCOLLOUGH

McCollough EG. The McCollough facial rejuvenation system: a condition-specific classification algorithm. Facial Plast Surg 2011;27(1):112–23.

McCollough EG, Perkins SW, Langsdon PR. SASMAS suspension rhytidectomy: rationale and long-term experience. Arch Otolaryngol Head Neck Surg 1989; 115:228–34.

REFERENCES: THOMAS

1. Perkins SW, Sandel HD. Chapter 35: Rhytidectomy. In: Thomas JR, editor. Advanced therapy in facial plastic & reconstructive surgery; 2010. p. 413–28.
2. Perkins SW, Patel AB. Extended superficial muscular aponeurotic system rhytidectomy: a graded approach. Facial Plast Surg Clin North Am 2009;17(4):57–87, vi.
3. Perkins SW, Koch BB. Simultaneous rhytidectomy and full-face carbon dioxide laser resurfacing: a case series and meta-analysis. Arch Facial Plast Surg 2002;4(4):227–33.
4. Thomas, Humphreys. Thomas procedures in facial plastic surgery. PMPH Publishing; 2011.
5. Zimbler, Kokoska, Thomas. Anatomy and pathophysiology of facial aging. Facial Plast Surg Clin North Am 2001;9(2).
6. Ivy, Lorenc, Aston. Plast Reconstr Surg 1996.

REFERENCES: PERKINS

7. Bassichis, Becker. Arch Facial Plast Surg 2004.
8. Tardy, Thomas. Facial aesthetic surgery. Mosby-Yearbook, Inc; 1995.
9. Thomas JR. Facial plastic surgery applications for liposuction. In: Cummings, editor. Otolaryngology-head and neck surgery. Mosby-Yearbook, Inc; 1990.
10. Mittelman H, Spencer JR, Chrzanowski DS. Chin region: management of grooves & mandibular hypoplasia with alloplastic implant. Facial Plast Surg Clin North Am 2007;15(4):445–60.
11. Ramirez OM. The subperiosteal rhytidectomy: the third generation facelift. Ann Plast Surg 1992;28:218–32.
12. McCollough EG, Perkins SW, Langsdon PR. SASMAS suspension rhytidectomy, rationale and long term experience. Arch Otolaryngol Head Neck Surg 1989;115:228–34.

13. Kamer FM. One hundred consecutive deep plane face lifts. Arch Otolaryngol Head Neck Surg 1996; 122:17–22.

14. Baker SR. Tri-plane rhytidectomy. Arch Otolaryngol Head Neck Surg 1997;123:1167–72.

15. Perkins SW, Williams JD, MacDonald K, et al. Prevention of seromas and hematomas after facelift surgery with the use of postoperative vacuum drains. Arch Otolaryngol Head Neck Surg 1997; 123:743–5.

Lip Augmentation
Discussion and Debate

Brian P. Maloney, MD[a],*, William Truswell IV, MD[b,c],*,
S. Randolph Waldman, MD[d],*

KEYWORDS

- Lip augmentation • Lip implants • Injectable fillers • Lip rejuvenation

---

Lip Augmentation Panel Discussion

Brian P. Maloney, William Truswell IV, and S. Randolph Waldman, address questions for discussion and debate:

1. Is surgery ever a better alternative than injectable fillers for enhancement of the lips?
2. What role do permanent lip implants play for today's patients?
3. How do you manage the small-mouthed person seeking lip enlargement?
4. How do you handle down-turning corners of the mouth?
5. How do you handle a person who previously had full lips but now is losing volume, especially in the corners?
6. What qualities of the lip are important to preserve when considering various lip augmentation materials and techniques?
7. What are the best ways of reducing the length of the upper lip?
8. *Analysis:* Over the past 5 years, how has your technique or approach to lips changed, or what is the most important thing you have learned in performing lip augmentations?

 Video of surgical technique of subnasal lip lift and advancement of lower lip accompanies this article. Available at: http://www.facialplastic.theclinics.com/

Is surgery ever a better alternative than injectable fillers for enhancement of the lips?

MALONEY

Yes, surgery may be a better alternative for the patient with thin lips and poor definition of Cupid's bow. For the patient with congenitally thin lips, the vermilion advancement is an excellent means of increasing the amount of vermilion show. This procedure can be combined with lip augmentation procedures if additional bulk is desired (**Fig. 1**).

Surgery is also an excellent procedure for the patient who desires lip augmentation; however,

---

[a] Maloney Center for Facial Plastic Surgery, 6111 Peachtree Dunwoody Road, Building E Suite 201, Atlanta, GA 30328, USA
[b] Private Practice, The University of Connecticut School of Medicine, Northampton, MA, USA
[c] Aesthetic Laser and Cosmetic Surgery Center, 61 Locust Street, Suite 2, Northampton, MA 01060, USA
[d] Waldman Plastic Surgery Center, 125 East Maxwell Street, Suite 303, Lexington, KY 40508, USA
* Corresponding authors.
E-mail addresses: faceinfo@bellsouth.net; bill.truswell@gmail.com; srwaldman@aol.com

Facial Plast Surg Clin N Am 20 (2012) 327–346
doi:10.1016/j.fsc.2012.05.003
1064-7406/12/$ – see front matter © 2012 Elsevier Inc. All rights reserved.

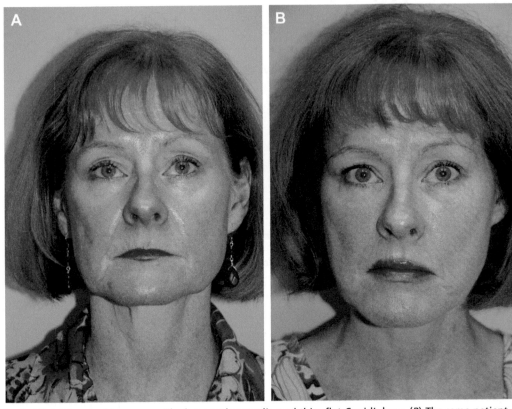

Fig. 1. (*A*) A 54-year-old woman with elongated upper lip and thin, flat Cupid's bow. (*B*) The same patient after upper-lip advancement and acellular dermal matrix augmentation of upper and lower lip. Injectable fillers would have lengthened an already long lip, not achieving the degree of vermilion show with the advancement.

the upper lip may be too long and the patient may display no incisor show. Augmenting the lips in this case would only make the lip longer, throwing the lips more out of balance. A nasal-base resection would be a better alternative to augmentation. Once the length of the lip is shortened, augmentation can be performed if necessary.

Acellular human dermal matrix graft augmentation of the lips can be an excellent means of creating more vermilion show in a thin-lipped patient. This surgical procedure is performed through a single incision in each commissure; a submucosal tunnel is created, and the matrix can be placed into both upper and lower lips.

When cosmetic surgeons attempt to create large lips from small ones by injecting fillers, the end result is generally a duck-bill, stiff, sausage-like look to the lip. The most commonly used lip fillers are hyaluronic acid fillers. By their physical nature they are liquids. Liquids by definition take the shape of their containers. It is very difficult to stretch a vermilion with a liquid filler and have it

result in a natural long-lasting change. With increasing refinements of hyaluronic acid, newer products offer a higher degree of cohesiveness. Cohesiveness refers to the molecules' ability to stay together and resist being dispersed. For high-motion areas that require augmentation, these highly cohesive fillers will offer more semi-solid properties; however, the end result of overfilling with the latest fillers generally is an overdramatic feature.

I have found multiple V-Y advancements of the entire wet lip surface as an augmentation technique to result in a bulky lip with poor movement. Lips are very dynamic in nature, and any surgical procedure needs to maintain a soft flexible lip to allow it to function properly. Man-made implants such as those using expanded polytetrafluoroethylene (ePTFE) and saline as fillers, tend in my experience to restrict lip movements and often result in extrusion when placed in the upper lip. The lower lip is more tolerant of the implants because of its more basic structure and movement.

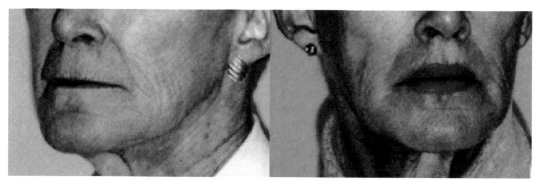

Fig. 2. Direct lift of upper and lower lip. Note shortening of the white upper lip.

TRUSWELL

Surgical lip enlargement should be considered in patients with very thin lips for whom injectable fillers or implants would be more distorting than enhancing. The best way to help these patients, in my opinion, is to perform a direct lip lift, a subnasal lip lift, or a V-Y augmentation. All of these procedures have varying results and can be fraught with complications.

Direct lip lifting is performed by excising a portion of the white lip and advancing the mucosa upward as an advancement flap. This technique will shorten the white upper lip. The incision should be placed above the white roll of the upper lip to preserve this feature. Meticulous closure is paramount in minimizing the scar that will occur. The patient must understand this issue. The scar can be camouflaged with dermabrasion or laser resurfacing. Lipstick can hide it, as can cosmetic tattoo. If not done with skill and precision, the scar can be emotionally and socially debilitating (**Figs. 2** and **3**).[6,9,10]

The subnasal lip lift is another technique designed to shorten the white lip while elevating the red lip. This procedure is done by excising a strip of skin with the incision placed just below and precisely following the gentle curve of the nasal sill. The remaining lip is elevated as an advancement flap and carefully sutured in place. Difficulties with this procedure include scar formation and the fact that this will only elevate the middle third of the upper lip.[6,9–11,24]

V-Y lip augmentation is a surgical approach that avoids skin incisions, therefore avoiding problems with cutaneous scarring. Good results require an exacting technique. Multiple V-Y flaps shift lateral tissues centrally to lift and add fullness to the lip. The lips can be projected forward by this technique, which can leave the patient with an unpleasant pucker. The thin, aged lip will not lend itself readily to this procedure. The postoperative course for this surgery can be prolonged, with considerable swelling and down-time for the patient.[1,2,4,8,9]

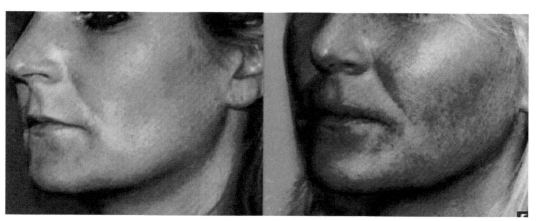

Fig. 3. Direct upper-lip lift (and rhinoplasty) 1 year postoperatively. Note faint scar at vermilion.

WALDMAN

Only in extreme situations and after lengthy conversation with the patient do we consider a surgical approach over the use of injectable fillers. Surgery is only appropriate for the rejuvenation patient who might present with increased distance between the vermilion and the base of the nose and also demonstrating loss of philtral architecture. In addition, there are situations whereby the corners of the mouth are so dependent that inject-able fillers have no chance at success. In this situation we may consider a corner-of-the-mouth lift. This operation has been well documented, as has the subnasal lip lift, in a previous issue of this journal. It is important to remember that there are specific indications and also anatomic prerequisites for either the subnasal lip lift or the corner-of-the-mouth lift. If these parameters are not present then surgery should not be considered.[1,2]

What role do permanent lip implants play for today's patients?

MALONEY

At this time, other than autologous fat or human acellular dermal matrix graft, I do not recommend "permanent lip implants." I have found that because of the high motion of the lip area, autologous fat may resorb. Success rates can be increased by asking the patient to limit lip movements for the first 2 weeks after the procedure to help with graft revascularization. In an unpublished multicenter study by Maloney, Waldman, and Kridel (1997), acellular dermal matrix grafts were found to result in lip augmentation for at least a year for 89% of the study patients.

Permanent injectable implants may include polymethylmethacrylate (PMMA) beads coated with cow collagen, or microdroplet silicone. Although the PMMA filler is on at least the third generation, I have seen so many reactions present from earlier generations that I do not consider it an option (**Fig. 4**). Multinucleated giant cells are known to surround both PMMA and microdroplet silicone. These cells may stay dormant for several years and then be activated. The end result can be swollen, red, tender nodules.

Over the years I have placed ePTFE lip implants in the upper and lower lips, only to see most of them extrude from the upper lip. I am concerned that recent modifications incorporating saline-filled lip implants would have the same result. This shortcoming is due to a basic difference between the embryology of the upper and lower lip, and their resultant movements. The upper lip flexes much more than the lower lip with speech, and therefore makes it less tolerant than the lower lip with regard to implants. I believe it is the complex movement of the lip as opposed to the configuration of the ePTFE that is the greatest challenge to be overcome with lip implants.

TRUSWELL

For some time now the public has shown an increasing desire for procedures that are quick

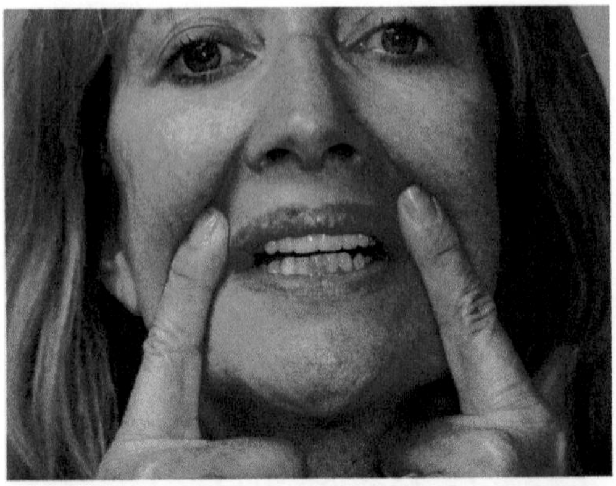

Fig. 4. A patient with extrusion of polymethylmetha-crylate beads. Notice the lumpy nature across the lip.

and affordable with the expenditure of no or minimal down-time. The results they seek are ones that are effective and long lasting, if not permanent.

One drawback of injectable fillers is that they are generally, in the short or long term, temporary with the exception of injectable silicon. The wish for a permanent solution has led to the development of soft-tissue implants. These materials include ePTFE, silicone gel, and silicon rubber (for nasolabial folds) among others. The ideal permanent implant will have the properties of ease of placement with little down-time, softness, no visibility, good biocompatibility and biointegration, no patient rejection, long-term predictability, minimal to no shrinkage, no migration, the ability to individualize the implant to the patient, ease of removal, and affordability. These attributes exist with the implants of ePTFE material.

The implants are not well suited for patients with very thin lips that have little vermilion showing. Otherwise they are an excellent choice for any patient wishing a permanent solution for lip augmentation. The implants insert readily with local anesthesia, and are soft and natural in appearance. The dual-porosity ePTFE implants have excellent biocompatibility and biointegration, allowing cellular ingrowth into the framework of the strands. These implants have little to no adverse effects on the motion and function of the lips and oral commissure, and do not alter the shape of the lips or mouth.[13,16,17] I have had extensive experience with dual-porosity ePTFE lip implants and have inserted more than 250 of them. I have had only one extruded, owing to infection. One patient had them replaced for shrinkage of less than 10% longitudinally. The implants are well tolerated and do not interfere with lip function, from whistling to kissing.

WALDMAN

Some physicians will use silastic implants to augment a younger person's lips. Such an approach is one we have not yet attempted, although we have not ruled it out should long-term results demonstrate patient satisfaction and minimal problems.

Previously we were among the first to use ePTFE for lip enhancement, but the material demonstrated too many variables in the healing process and we abandoned this procedure in favor of the new improved group of temporary injectable fillers. Other materials that have been tried but have not stood the test of time include cadaver dermis, dermal-fat grafts, and injectable silicone. In general, however, I would say that whatever we use in the lips must be easily reversible, that is, no residual damage to the lips following removal!

Remember the phrase on many of our diplomas that reminds us "Physician first do no harm." Too often we forget this as aesthetic plastic surgeons.

How do you manage the small-mouthed person seeking lip enlargement?

MALONEY

Beauty by definition is a face that is in proportion and balance. Surgically creating a larger mouth can be challenging. Therefore, I begin my physical examination by evaluating the patient's overall facial proportions. If the lower third of the face has squared off because of excess facial fat or ptosis of the cheek fat pad caused by aging, the mouth will appear smaller. For the most patients as they age, the ratio of the width of the face to the width of the mouth increases. If the face can be narrowed by facial liposuction or a facelift, I will discuss these options with the patient. If a patient has thick facial skin, I may also discuss partial or total removal of the buccal fat pad in an attempt to narrow the width of the face (**Fig. 5**).

If a patient with a small mouth has an overprojecting chin, this should be addressed with the patient. A reverse genioplasty or burring down of a prominent pogonion will help to reduce the size of the inferior border of the face.

If the lips are thin and have poor definition of Cupid's bow, a vermilion advancement will help to increase the amount of vermilion show. The lateral extent of the incisions can come within a few millimeters of the commissure, but never extend beyond or to the commissure. The advancement can be combined with lip augmentation procedures to increase the bulk of the lips. Care should be exercised not to overfill the central portion of the lip, as

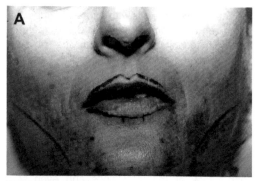

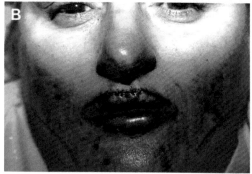

Fig. 5. (*A*) A patient with small mouth relative to facial width. Markings show planned facial liposuction and removal of buccal fat pad, and upper and lower lip advancement. (*B*) The same patient following these procedures. Notice the increased size of the mouth, relative to the width of the face.

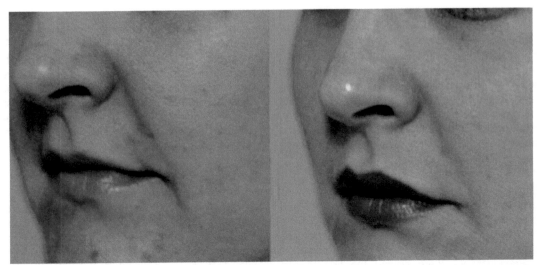

Fig. 6. Preoperative and 6-month postoperative views of small "cupie doll" mouth with 3 implants in the upper lip.

this will highlight the small nature of the mouth. Augmentation should focus on creating a smooth even lip from commissure to commissure.

TRUSWELL

The patient who presents with a small or "cupie doll" mouth requires some thought and consideration. Whatever technique is selected, the physician must take care not to overenhance the lips. Injectable fillers in excess will easily lend a duck-bill look

WALDMAN

We use a very conservative approach to the use of filler injections. Large lips in this scenario will appear too artificial. We also avoid anything that might change the general shape of the lips. All too often when I look at the magazines and even some presentations, I see that the lateral portion of the lips is out of proportion to the central area. Some-

I have seen some patients undergo permanent lip tattooing, with moderate success, to create the illusion of a larger mouth.

to the lips. Surgical enhancement such as the V-Y mucosal approach can produce a fish-mouth appearance. The ePTFE soft-tissue implants work quite well, retaining the same natural shape and look of the mouth without distortion (**Fig. 6**).

times this is severe enough that it appears the patient might have a "whistler's deformity," which to me is very unnatural. Another common mistake is to create upper lip dominance (often described by my patients as the "Howard the Duck" look) when in nature the lower lip is almost always slightly larger and more voluminous than the upper lip.

How do you handle down-turning corners of the mouth?

MALONEY

Few other facial features impart such negative connotations as the down-turning corner of the mouth. The implications are of frequent frowning, scowling, and generalized unhappiness. In reality, the marionette lines, as they are frequently called, may develop for most of us while we sleep. It is uncertain as to the percentage of people who grind or clench their teeth at night, but it is very high. While the masseter is working away grinding

the teeth, the depressor anguli oris (DAO) is also at work. This frequent action of the muscle wears away the soft tissues in the area, resulting in the deepening groove. Other facial components playing a role in developing a down-turning mouth are relaxation of the cheek skin, contributing to the jowl, loss of vertical dental height, and loss of vermilion volume. The down-turning mouth is a gradual process. Therefore, patients present

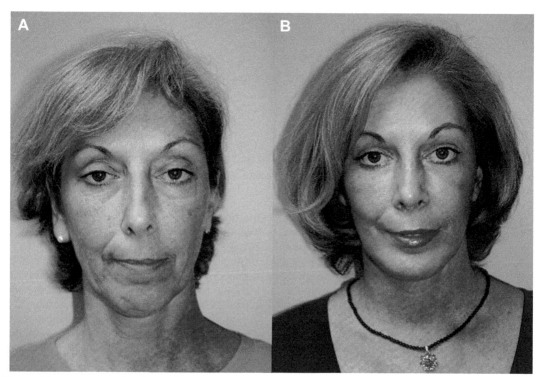

Fig. 7. (A) A patient with advanced down-turning of the mouth down to the mandible. (B) Elevation of the corner of the mouth achieved with extended chin implant, autologous fat transfer, and facelift to soften the jowl component.

with a spectrum ranging from early down-turning of the corner to full-blown loss of volume from the corner down to the mandibular edge.

For the patient with early down-turning corners of the mouth, botulinum toxin injections to the DAO may be all that is required. I generally place 2 units of onabotulinum toxin, a centimeter lateral and a centimeter inferior to the commissure. Care should be exercised, if placing toxin, at the inferior aspect of the DAO. The origin of the DAO overlaps the origin of the depressor labii inferioris (DLI) on the lateral surface of the mandible. If the botulinum toxin affects the DLI, the patient will notice that the lip on that side will be elevated.

As the down-turning corner advances down toward the mandible, volume is necessary to help restore a more youthful contour. Hyaluronic acid fillers can be placed along the fold in an office setting. When dealing with patients with a down-turning corner of the mouth, the filler is generally added in combination with the botulinum toxin. In mild cases, I prefer to place the hyaluronic acid

injections in a cross-hatching pattern at the corner of the mouth, in a subcutaneous plane, to help support this dynamic area. In more advanced cases, where the tissue has melted away after years of use down to the mandibular margin, I prefer to start at the mandible and work superiorly.

In the setting of an operating room, I prefer autologous fat for filling, placed in a similar fashion as already described. If a patient has microgenia, an extended chin implant that wraps around the anterior mandibular angle can be combined with the fat to help strengthen the area. Although a facelift procedure may soften the jowl component of down-turning corner of the mouth, it should not be viewed as a sole treatment for the area. The facelift is generally combined with the necessary aforementioned procedures to collectively soften the down-turning corner in the mature patient (**Fig. 7**).

I have never seen a corner lip lift that I considered aesthetically pleasing. This technique of surgically excising a triangle of skin at the corner has left patients with more of a "Joker" look.

TRUSWELL

There is no perfect remedy to correct the down-turning of the corners of the mouth. It is one of the truly frustrating aging signs that facial plastic

surgeons deal with. Many different techniques are used to soften and correct this defect, including injectable fillers, chemodenervation,

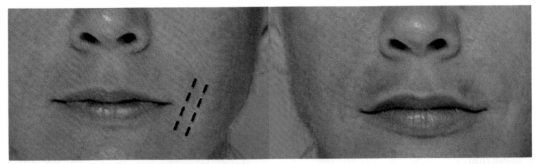

Fig. 8. Views pretreatment and 1 week after hyaluronic acid injections to upper and lower lips and obliquely lateral to the commissures. Note corner of mouth lift.

and surgery. The cause of the downturn occurs because of different factors. The DAO exerts a downward pull on the corners, loss of volume accentuates the appearance, and descent of the jowl further defines the problem. One, two, or all of the problems may need to be addressed in any given patient.

A simple technique that gives reliable results is the use of hydroxyapatite. Two linear injections of about 0.15 mL of this filler are placed parallel to one another. The first is injected 1 mm lateral to the oral commissure. It is placed 45° obliquely to a horizontal line drawn between the lips when closed and oriented outward toward the ear. A tiny bolus is deposited at the level of the commissure as the needle is withdrawn. The second injection is 3 to 4 mm lateral and parallel to the first, affording a slight lift to the corner of the mouth. Additional filler can be used to enhance the marionette line if necessary (**Fig. 8**).

Chemodenervation with Botox or Dysport can be used to immobilize the lip depressor. The unopposed action and tone of the levator muscles will raise the commissure. With the patient frowning the depressor can be palpated inferolaterally to

the commissure, and sometimes it can be seen. Two to 3 mL of the agent is injected into the bulk of the muscle.

Surgical elevation of the corners is another approach to this problem. This procedure involves excising a triangle of skin above the corner of the mouth and lifting the commissure in closure. A line is marked from the corner medially along the vermilion for 1 to 1.5 cm. A second line is marked from the corner for the same distance on a trajectory toward the top of the tragus. A curvilinear line 7 to 9 mm above their junction connects the upper ends of each line. This area to be excised will look like a baseball diamond. The skin is excised and after hemostasis, the wound is approximated in appropriate fashion. The downsides to this procedure are the permanent scars that will need camouflage, and there will be an unacceptable smirk to the mouth if too much skin has been excised.[22]

That there are several approaches to this problem strengthens the argument that no single technique is ideal. It may also be necessary to perform a facelift to aid in the heavily jowled individual.

WALDMAN

Again, as for the small-mouthed person, we prefer injectable fillers for this concern with down-turning corners of the mouth. Multiple treatments over a long period of time may be very helpful. Of course, facelifting can also provide some

improvement. In extreme situations we consider the corner-of-the-mouth lift. Extreme problems with the commissure downturn can even lead to chronic drooling, and secondary irritant or even fungal dermatitis.

How do you handle a person who previously had full lips but now is losing volume, especially in the corners?

MALONEY

The patient who previously had full lips but over time has lost volume is generally an ideal one for lip augmentation. I generally prefer a hyaluronic acid filler for in-office correction. If the

patient is going to the operating room for another reason, I will generally recommend placing autologous fat in the lip and perioral area.

The challenging part of this question is the revolumizing of the lateral corners of the lips, which tend to disappear first. This condition is not only a reflection of loss of vermilion volume but also changes in the surrounding soft tissues, facial bones, and tooth position and length. The patient's physical examination will often reveal which components are contributory. Tooth position and anatomy play a large role in lip aesthetics. If the teeth have had significant loss, vertical lengthening, or malposition, dental restoration may be indicated.

Loss of lateral lip volume may be the earliest sign of the beginning of the down-turning of the corner of the mouth. Treatment options for a hyperactive DAO muscle should be followed as discussed in the previous section. If the patient has experienced lengthening of the lip, a lip-shortening procedure may be indicated.

Technically, I have found that placing the hyaluronic acid filler along the anterior aspect of the lip and then making a second pass on the inside of the wet line of the lip may help to roll the lip out to the patient's satisfaction.

TRUSWELL

Volume loss of the pink lip occurs with age and can have an unpleasant effect on one's countenance. In general, men have thinner lips than women. With age, the faces of women become more masculine. Men have lower, flatter eyebrows, squarer jaws, heavier necks, coarser skin, and thinner lips. Thin lips can convey the appearance of anger, meanness, or parsimony. As for all the attributes that we wish to improve in the lips, there is no single solution for loss of volume in the corners. Lip advancement procedures, implants, and fillers can all help to varying degrees.

I believe that the hyaluronic acid injectable fillers are the best solution to this problem. While soft-tissue implants certainly add volume, the corners of the mouth are least affected. I often will use the injectable filler in the lip corners with the permanent implants in place to restore volume in this spot.

Surgical techniques, direct lip lifts, and corner-of-the-mouth lifts will increase the vertical height of the lip. However, the pink lip will look flat in many instances. Here, as well, it may be desirable to combine the surgery with injectable filler.

WALDMAN

Again, this is a perfect scenario for the use of injectable fillers. I use Perlane for shaping and Juvederm for plumping. Also, in this scenario it is important to consider plumping of the white upper lip region to eliminate vertical rhytids and also to recreate the philtral architecture. Remember what has been mentioned earlier about avoiding upper lip dominance, especially on the profile view. This look is one that makes patients absolutely cringe!

What qualities of the lip are important to preserve when considering various lip augmentation materials and techniques?

MALONEY

The lips are not only a central aesthetic feature of the face, they perform many roles; lip movements contribute to speech, act as a sphincter when eating and drinking, and act as a sensory organ with kissing. Most patients may temporarily experience some numbness or tightness following lip procedures. As a general rule the greater the augmentation, the longer the recovery for the patient. At the end of the healing period it is important that the lips need to remain, soft, flexible, and mobile.

From a technical perspective, the design of the procedure and implant choices may influence these qualities. I generally prefer to make a single incision in the commissure when placing acellular dermis in the lips. I have seen surgeons make 4 incisions to accomplish the same result. To me this seems to create additional scarring, which could restrict lip function.

The choice of filler is also very important for long-term success. Surgeons often focus on the here and now. It is important to look at patients from a long-term perspective. If a filler generates a lot of tissue response, over time the patient may experience tightening or limitation of movement of the lips. When this occurs, future lip procedures may become complicated or impossible to perform.

TRUSWELL

There are many physical attributes that must be considered when recommending and planning lip augmentation. Ideal proportions of the lips and perioral region in full-face view will show the upper one-third of the area includes the pink and white portions from the nasal sill to the center of the lower edge of the pink lip. The lower two-thirds encompass the lower lip to the bottom of the chin. The length of the lips from corner to corner should match the distance between the medial limbi of the irises. On lateral view, the upper and lower lips when closed should extend beyond a vertical line drawn from the subnasale to the pogonion. The upper lip should project between 2 and 3 mm more than the lower. The chin should sit within 1 mm of a line dropped from the vermilion-skin junction of the lower lip in the horizontal Frankfort plane.

The vermilion of the upper lip rises from the commissures to Cupid's bow. The apices of this landmark meet the lower ends of the philtral ridges. The white roll defines the border between the pink of the mucosa and the white

of the skin. It is important to not distort or ablate these areas with any procedure performed on the lips.[23]

Other qualities to evaluate in the aging lip include the mucosal surface. It should be determined whether there are any lesions, venous lakes, or areas of cheilitis. The skin also must be assessed. Identify the skin type, presence of lesions, sun damage, rhytides, and traumatic or acne scars.

The needs and desires of the patient must be assessed with respect to lifestyle as well as self-image. Altered sensation may accompany lip augmentation and could negatively affect such activities as kissing and instrumental horn playing. Some individuals exercise various characteristics of facial motion in verbal communication that become part of their personae. If these are altered by any technique performed, it may have a devastating effect on self-image. The facial plastic surgeon must understand that once the initial thrill of more attractive lips has waned, regrets may be felt for unique personal traits lost.[1]

WALDMAN

I am always concerned about the appearance of the philtral area or Cupid's bow. It is also important regarding what I have emphasized in the preceding discussions. We almost always treat both the upper and lower lip. It is also rare for us to use more than one syringe during any single

session. If patients want more, we will have them return in 3 weeks for a second session. With today's fillers it is easy to create unnatural-appearing lips when injecting too much. I also use only hyaluronic acid fillers in the lips because they are easily reversible.

What are the best ways of reducing the length of the upper lip?

MALONEY

A long upper lip may be congenital or more commonly acquired. If the patient has a long upper lip with a well-defined Cupid's bow, a nasal-base resection of skin can help to restore proportion to the lip area. The amount of skin to excise can be calculated by measuring the thirds of the face, and dividing by two-thirds. The difference between the actual length of the upper lip and the ideal length is the amount of skin to be excised. The skin is outlined in a gull-wing fashion following the nasal base, and excised in a full-thickness fashion (**Fig. 9**). The incision generally heals well. If the incision has not healed to the patient's satisfaction, dermabrasion can be used to help improve the appearance of the scar.

The other common long-lip scenario is when a patient has a poorly defined Cupid's bow area. In these patients vermilion advancement may be

preferred (see **Fig. 1**). Patients will have to weigh the pros and cons of the various scar locations along the nasal base or vermilion margin. With lip advancements, the ellipse of skin to be excised is agreed on by both the patient and surgeon. Technically the challenge is to stabilize the lips to allow a clean incision; this can be performed by applying downward pressure at each commissure to stabilize the lip on the underlying teeth. This procedure is particularly helpful in an older patient with thin lip. A younger patient with more lip mass may require less stabilization.

When making the incision, care must be taken to bevel the edges of the incision. The depth of the incision is just through the dermis; care should be taken to minimize damage to the underlying muscle. Meticulous wound eversion with closure completes the surgical steps a surgeon may follow

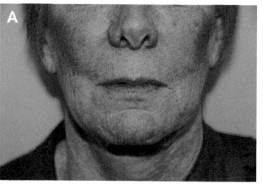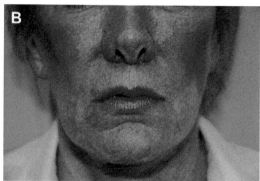

Fig. 9. (A) A patient with a long, thin upper lip and moderate Cupid's bow definition. (B) The same patient following nasal base resection and hyaluronic acid lip augmentation.

to increase success. Postoperative instructions include resting the lips for 2 weeks and avoiding pulling or stretching of the mouth area for 6 weeks, to help minimize excessive strain on the incision. Botulinum toxin can be placed at several points just above the vermilion-cutaneous junction to further help rest the area. Excessive pulling can result in hypertrophy of the scar. If the scar hypertrophies, monthly injections of a dilute steroid injection are performed until the situation resolves.

Education of the patient regarding minimizing any excessive stretching of the healing lips is important to help prevent hypertrophy of the lip scar. Patients generally can cover the vermilion-cutaneous junction scar with lipstick to camouflage it. If necessary, permanent cosmetics can be placed into the lip and scar to help achieve a more finished look.

While either nasal base resection or vermilion advancement can be performed in men, often electrolysis is necessary postoperatively. Especially with the vermilion advancement, an experienced electrologist needs to remove a 2- to 3-mm wide strip around the perimeter of the lip to help create a white-roll look.

TRUSWELL

Options to reduce the length of the lip are limited. As the face ages, the white lip lengthens in proportion to and as a result of shrinkage of the pink lip. Visually, lipstick or tattoo can be applied above the vermilion to change the proportion. However, this most often appears false and unattractive. Augmentation procedures of the pink lip will, likewise, change the ratio of pink-lip length to white-lip length. The best method, in my opinion, is surgical alteration. Direct lip lifting will lengthen the pink lip and shorten the white lip. However, the white roll will appear attenuated and a visible scar will result (Fig. 10). The subnasal lip lift is the best approach. This lift will also produce a scar, but it will be hidden by the shadow of the nose. This procedure will lift the middle third of the upper lip. The incision is placed within 2 mm of the nasal sill, carefully following the curved contour. The skin is undermined and one-third to as much as one-half is excised. Closure is meticulous.[5,9,24]

WALDMAN

At times, use of injectable fillers to provide curvature of the lip will result in a shorter-appearing lip; however, injecting volume into the vermilion of the upper lip itself can make the lip look even longer and result in additional hooding of the upper dentition when talking or smiling. In the older patient, as mentioned in the first question of this discussion, we consider the subnasal lip lift with possible use of vermilion filler injections as a secondary procedure (Fig. 11). Many times when we perform the subnasal lip lift we will also perform a vermilion advancement of the lower lip. See Video of surgical technique of subnasal lip lift with advancement of lower lip. It is very rare for me to consider vermilion advancement of the upper lip, however, as the scar is more of a potential concern in that area.[1,2]

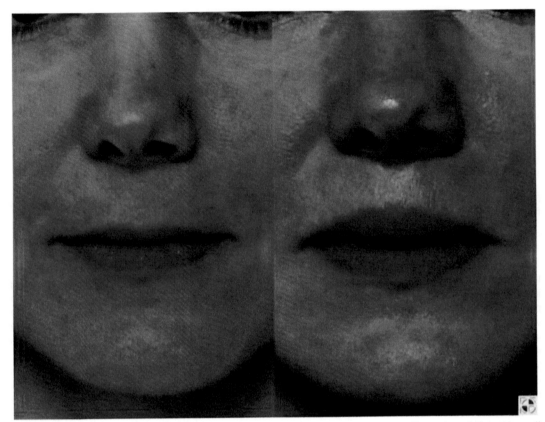

Fig. 10. Preoperative and 3-month postoperative views of direct upper-lip lift. Note flattening of the white roll, a very minimal scar, and shortening of the white lip.

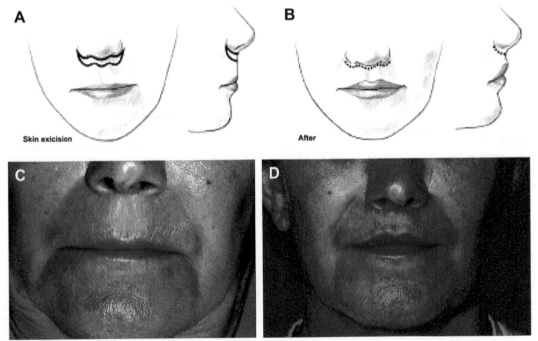

Fig. 11. Effect on lips of subnasal lip lift. (*A, C*) preoperative, (*B, D*) postoperative. (*From* Waldman R. The subnasal lip lift. Facial Plast Surg Clin North Am 2007;15:513–6; with permission.)

Analysis: Over the past 5 years, how has your technique or approach to lips changed, or what is the most important thing you have learned in performing lip augmentations?

MALONEY

Most fields of aesthetic medicine have undergone significant advances over the past 10 years; however, the lip area continues to be a challenging area for most doctors. In my practice, I believe lip augmentation procedures have improved as a result of my better understanding of the embryology, lip dynamics, perioral aging, and implant advancements.

Having incorporated these different concepts into my evaluation causes me to look at lips as a regional structure instead of as an isolated feature. The first portion of this discussion focuses on some of these areas and how they have shaped my approach to lip surgery.

Knowledge of the developmental anatomy of the lips is the foundation for understanding the functional properties of the lips and the limitations they may place on surgical options. The upper lip forms from a condensation of 2 lateral subunits and a central unit. The end result of this fusion is a unique structure characterized by the philtral ridges, philtral sulcus, and Cupid's bow. The lower lip forms from the fusion of 2 components, which is why the lower lip does not have a Cupid's bow or ridges.

Because of the different embryologic development, the upper and lower lips function very differently. The upper lip flexes much more than the lower during speech. These differences in movement place different stresses on the upper lip, and therefore make it less tolerant to procedures that restrict its movement.

Aesthetic treatment of the lips has changed from a localized structural approach to more of a regional treatment approach. A regional approach to cosmetic lip surgery allows the surgeon to take a step back and view the whole picture; that is, viewing a painting as a whole instead of focusing on one feature of the painting. This approach has led to improved cosmetic results because there are so many factors coming into play in this area. As the face ages, the height of the teeth decreases, and the face begins to turn inward, the bones of the face begin to lose volume, the skin begins to relax causing flattening and blunting of Cupid's bow, and vermilion volume decreases. It is important for the surgeon to assess all of these structures during the physical examination. When consulting more mature patients, having an opportunity to review photographs from when they were younger can be very helpful in understanding some of the changes that have taken place over time. I generally recommend that patients bring in photographs taken when they were in their twenties. My personal feeling is that this is when the lips' volume and facial structures are at their aesthetic peak for most patients. The photographs can also be used to discuss with the patient what changes may be possible and which ones may not be addressed.

The patient consultation regarding lip procedures is an important meeting, where the patient's goals and aesthetic taste are discussed. Every surgeon has a different aesthetic sense, and patients similarly vary in their concept of an ideal look. During the consultation, photographs of previous patients or magazine photographs can help the physician and patient arrive at a meeting of the minds. If common ground is not found, it may be best not to accept the patient into one's practice. Frequently I turn away patients who desire large, unnatural lips.

TRUSWELL

Many techniques and approaches to lip augmentation have evolved over many years. Their popularity has waxed and waned. There is still no true consensus as to the best method. Today the filler companies market directly to patients, and this has driven the demand for specific products in their direction. Are the different available hyaluronic acid products significantly different from one another? I think not. I have evolved my approach to lip augmentation over the years by my own experience and to some degree by patient demand.

The techniques used today include direct surgery,[3,8–11] permanent, semipermanent, and temporary injectable fillers,[9,11–15] and soft-tissue implants.[16–18] Selection of technique for any given patient requires careful assessment of the specific problem at hand. Attributes that must be analyzed include the proportion of white to pink lip, lip volume, the degree or relative absence of Cupid's bow, down-turning of the corners of the mouth, the condition of the mucosa, and the presence and degree of rhytides and solar changes in the perioral skin.[5,7,9]

It is important to analyze the situation at hand and the needs and desires of the patient when deciding on an approach. Permanent implants are just that. What may be wonderful in the eyes of the patient today may be inappropriate decades hence. Complications of permanent implants include infection, extrusion, asymmetry, shrinkage, lip bowing, migration, visibility on movement, and hardness.[16] Some, ePTFE, are readily removable whereas others, liquid silicon, are at best difficult if not impossible to remove. Temporary injectables need to be repeated to maintain the enhancement. Semipermanent injectable materials have been associated with granuloma formation.[9,12] Direct surgery can result in troublesome scar formation. A combination of procedures may be needed to correct the problem, for example surgical lip lengthening and volume enhancement. Lip augmentation may interfere with some lip functions such as whistling, horn blowing, using a straw, and kissing.

Taking all of the aforesaid into consideration, the procedure I prefer for lip augmentation as an isolated procedure is the insertion of dual-porosity ePTFE soft-tissue implants. Many patients prefer a permanent implant to avoid repeated costs and repeated procedures. ePTFE has been used successfully as an implant material for many years.[16,17,19,20] It is safe, biocompatible, and inert. The initial use of ePTFE implants was complicated by a high incidence of shrinkage and hardness, because of the low porosity of the ePTFE implants as first used. These original implants had an internodal distance of 30 μm, which prevents biointegration of the embedded tissue, producing a fibrous capsule and allowing migration. With time, the capsule tends to contract and shrink the implant. The dual-porosity implants were developed about 12 years ago to lessen this problem. The surface of the new implants has an internodal distance of 40 μm, which is porous enough to allow limited radial biointegration, thus limiting capsule formation and preventing migration. The inner core, exposed on the ends, has an internodal distance of 100 μm (**Fig. 12**), making a very soft implant, and the end exposure allows greater longitudinal biointegration. If necessary, these are easily removed.[16]

I prefer to inject the patient's lips with a hyaluronic acid filler before placing the permanent implant, thus allowing the patient and myself to determine what size best suits her needs and preferences. It also allows her some time to decide whether she likes the enhancement enough to proceed with the implant. The surgery is performed when the injectable fades away.

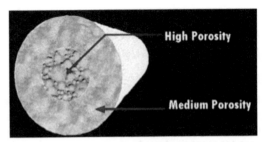

Fig. 12. Cross-section dual-porosity expanded polytetrafluoroethylene soft-tissue implant.

The implants are available as strands both round and oval in cross-sectional shape. I prefer the oval shape. For the upper lip, I use 2 pieces at the vermilion, because crossing Cupid's bow produces a "bowstring" effect on animation and stiffens the upper lip, inhibiting motion. I use one continuous piece from commissure to commissure across the lower lip. The long axis of the oval is oriented vertically, which raises the upper lip and provides a pout. For greater enhancement, I will add a third piece to the upper lip (second to the lower) at the wet-dry line with the long axis of the oval oriented obliquely outward with respect to each lip. This added piece starts 5 to 8 mm medial to the commissures. I have designed an insertion instrument (the Truswell Insertion Instrument; Marina Medical, Sunrise, FL, USA) (**Fig. 13**) to facilitate the implant placement. It consists of a solid handle with a detachable hollow shaft. A trocar, 4.0 mm and 6.0 mm in diameter, slides into the shaft and locks into the handle. It comes with an alligator forceps. The procedure is usually done with local anesthesia as a stand-alone procedure.

The face is prepped with an antiseptic solution and sterilely draped. Anesthesia is obtained by blocking the infraorbital and mandibular nerves with and local infiltration of 1% lidocaine with

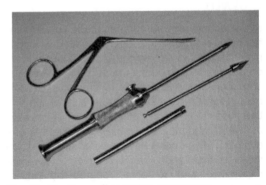

Fig. 13. The Truswell Insertion Instrument.

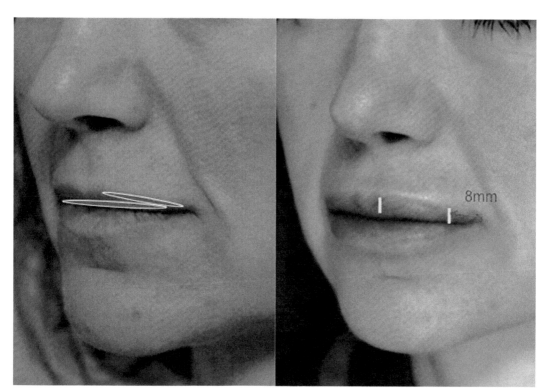

Fig. 14. (*Left*) Placement of left implant at vermilion and location of third implant at the wet-dry line for a fuller lip. (*Right*) Placement of incisions for 3 implants in the upper lip.

1:1000 epinephrine. After 10 minutes, vertical 3-mm incisions are made at the commissures on the vermilion of the lip (or 5–8 mm medial to the commissures if the added pieces are used) and beneath the peaks of the lip at Cupid's bow. The insertion instrument is passed from the lateral incision out through the medial incision (or corner to corner on the lower lip). The trocar is released and removed from the shaft. The alligator forceps is inserted into the shaft of the instrument, and the handle and shaft are removed from the wound. The forceps is now through the created tunnel. I taper one end of the ePTFE strand, grasp it with the forceps, and draw it through the tunnel and out from the incision. I have the patient open her mouth wide and I manually stretch the lip over the implant. Each end is then trimmed, beveled, and tapered, and inserted under the mucosa. The wounds are closed with a single horizontal mattress suture of 6-0 plain gut, slightly pursing the edges (**Figs. 14–16**).[13,17]

The patients are given a prescription for a cephalosporin, if not allergic, and are instructed to ice as much as possible for several days and to minimize facial expressions for 3 weeks. Acetaminophen is sufficient for analgesia. The patients are instructed that the implants will be manually palpable, although the degree of palpation lessens over time as biointegration ensues.

In 2003, a 5-physician multicenter retrospective study was presented at the Annual Meeting of the American Academy of Facial Plastic and Reconstructive Surgery. This study reported on a 30-month experience of 526 implants placed in

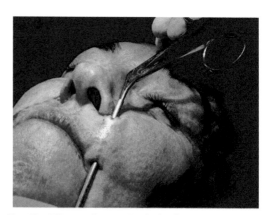

Fig. 15. Alligator forceps in shaft of Truswell Insertion Instrument in nasolabial fold.

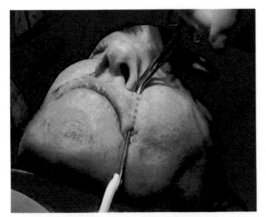

Fig. 16. Alligator forceps grasping implant before drawing it into place.

the lips, nasolabial folds, and marionette lines of 261 patients. The combined shrinkage rate was 3%, the combined infection rate 4%, and the patient satisfaction rate, satisfied and very satisfied, was 90%.[21]

As of 2010 I have inserted more than 250 dual-porosity ePTFE soft-tissue implants in lips. All but 2 patients were women. One patient developed an infection, and required implant removal and reinsertion 3 weeks later. One patient decided a year later that she no longer wanted a "foreign substance" in her lips and requested removal. No patient complained of impaired lip function. In particular, kissing was not impaired, as attested to by many patients and their partners. One patient experienced a longitudinal shrinkage, and requested and received a new implant. The degree of shrinkage was less than 10% in length. Today, industry and peer experience drives patients to request certain procedures and products in medicine and especially in cosmetic facial surgery. Injectable fillers are the most sought-after solution for lip enhancement by patients. That said, it is the physician's duty to educate the patient in all the available options so that the patient can make an informed choice. The safety, outcomes, patient satisfaction, and permanence of the dual-porosity soft-tissue implants make this procedure an excellent option for lip augmentation (**Figs. 17–21**).

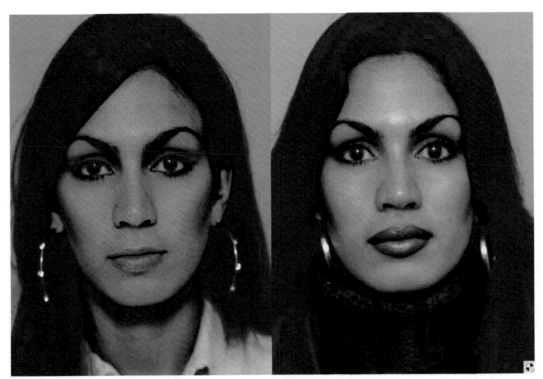

Fig. 17. A 25-year-old model. (*Left*) Preoperative view shows thin upper lip and full lower lip. (*Right*) Six-month postoperative view, after 3 soft-tissue implants were placed in the upper lip.

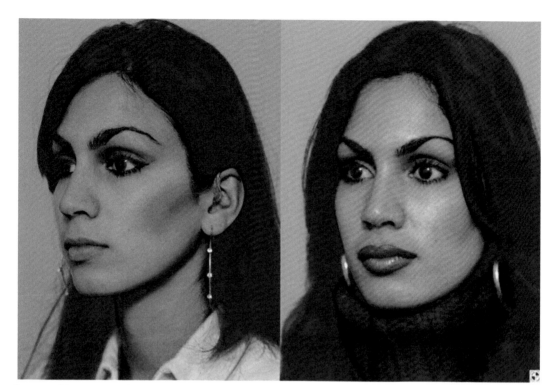

Fig. 18. Oblique view of the patient in **Fig. 17.**

WALDMAN

I am much more conservative in the amount of filler material that I use in any single session. I never inject more than 1 mL of any material into the lip.

I use one product to outline the lips and one product to plump the lips, but when called on to do both I will stage the procedure a couple of weeks apart. We often treat vertical lines involving the white portion of the upper lip with a horizontal filling technique, and rarely inject vertical lines in a vertical fashion. We often combine this with

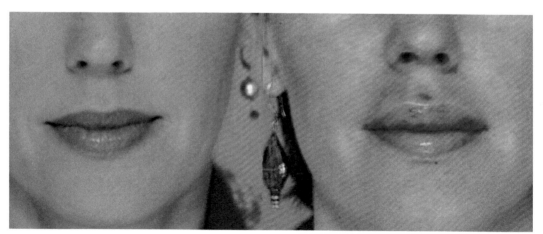

Fig. 19. Preoperative and 1-week postoperative views, showing the upper lip with 3 implants (2 at the vermilion and one at the wet-dry line) and the lower lip with one implant at the wet-dry line.

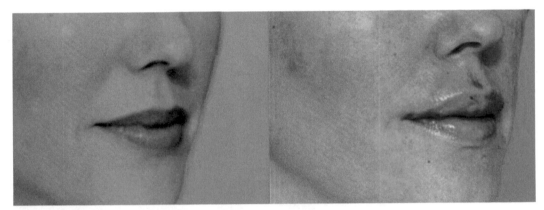

Fig. 20. Oblique view of the patient in **Fig. 19.**

phenol/croton oil chemical peeling to further rejuvenate the white portion of the upper lip.

Also, I do not use permanent materials of any kind in the lip, and we limit the 3 surgical approaches to lip enhancement to the rare rejuvenation patient who demonstrates clear and apparent indications:

1. Lip lift
2. Lip advancement
3. Corner-of-the-mouth lift.

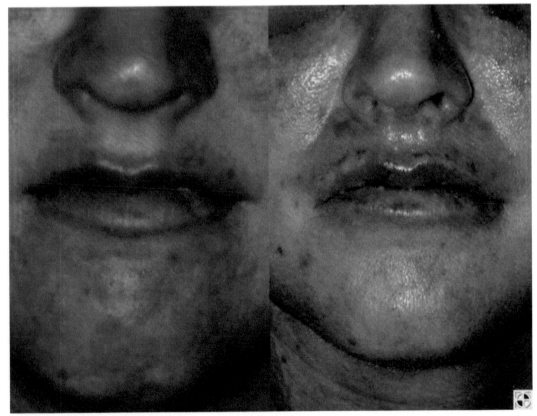

Fig. 21. Preoperative and 1-week postoperative views of a patient with 2 implants at vermilion border of the upper lip and laser resurfacing of the upper lip.

SUPPLEMENTARY DATA

Supplementary data related to this article can be found online at http://dx.doi.org/10.1016/j.fsc.2012.05.003.

SUGGESTED READINGS: MALONEY

Carlotti A, Aschaffenburg P, Schendel S. Facial changes associated with surgical advancement of the lip and maxilla. J Oral Maxillofac Surg 2010;44(8):593–6.

Fulton J, Rahimi D, Helton P, et al. Lip rejuvenation. Dermatol Surg 2001;26(5):470–6.

Gatti J. Permanent lip augmentation with serial fat grafting. Ann Plast Surg 1999;42(4):102–11.

Jacono A, Quatela V. Quantitative analysis of lip appearance After V-Y lip augmentation. Arch Facial Plast Surg 2004;6(3):172–7.

Kanchwala S, Bucky L. Facial fat grafting: the search for predictable results. Facial Plast Surg 2003;19(1):137–46.

Linder R. Permanent lip augmentation employing polytetrafluoroethylene grafts. Plast Reconstr Surg 1992;90(6):1083–90.

Maloney BP. Aesthetic surgery of the lip. In: Papel ID, Frodel J, Holt GR, et al, editors. Facial plastic and reconstructive surgery. 3rd edition. New York: Thieme; 2009. p. 459–68.

McCollough EG, Maloney BP. Aesthetic lip advancement. Am J Cosmet Surg 1996;13:207–12.

Monheit G, Coleman K. Hyaluronic acid fillers. Dermatol Ther 2006;19(3):141–50.

Moore K. The developing human. Philadelphia: W.B.Saunders; 1977. p. 156–74.

O'Conner GB. Surgical formation of the philtrum and the cutaneous upsweep. Am J Cosmet Surg 1958;95:227–30.

REFERENCES: TRUSWELL

1. Keller G. Considerations in V-Y lip augmentation. Arch Facial Plast Surg 2004;6:179.

2. Jacono AA. A new classification of lip zones to customize injectable lip augmentation. Arch Facial Plast Surg 2008;10(1):25–9.

3. Agarwal A, Gracely E, Maloney RW. Lip augmentation using sternocleidomastoid muscle and fascia grafts. Arch Facial Plast Surg 2010;12(2):97–102.

4. Truswell WH. Toward an ideal lip augmentation procedure. Arch Facial Plast Surg 2004;6:178.

5. Ali MJ, Ende K, Maas CS. Perioral rejuvenation and lip augmentation. Facial Plast Surg Clin North Am 2007;15(4):491–500.

6. Maloney BP. Aesthetic surgery of the lip. In: Papel ID, editor. Facial plastic and reconstructive surgery. 2nd edition. New York: Thieme Medical Publishers; 2002. p. 344–52.

7. Papel ID, Hill LE. Evaluation of the aging face. In: William H, Truswell IV, editors. Surgical facial rejuvenation; a road map to safe and reliable outcomes. New York: Thieme Medical Publishers; 2009. p. 1–8.

8. Jacono AA, Quatela VC. Quantitative analysis of lip appearance after V-Y lip augmentation. Arch Facial Plast Surg 2004;6:172–7.

9. Segall L, Ellis D. Therapeutic options for lip augmentation. Facial Plast Surg Clin North Am 2007;15(4):485–90.

10. Fanous N. Correction of thin lips: "lip lift". Plast Reconstr Surg 1984;74:33–41.

11. Waldman SR. The subnasal lip lift. Facial Plast Surg Clin North Am 1997;5:65–70.

12. Barnett JG, Barnett CR. Silicone augmentation of the lip. Facial Plast Surg Clin North Am 2007;15(4):501–12.

13. Truswell WH. Using permanent implant materials for cosmetic enhancement of the perioral region. Facial Plast Surg Clin North Am 2007;15(4):433–44.

14. Von Buelow S, Pallua N. Efficacy and safety of polyacrylamide hydrogel for facial soft tissue augmentation in a 2 year follow-up: a prospective multicenter study for evaluation of safety and aesthetic results in 101 patients. Plast Reconstr Surg 2006;118(3S):85S–91S.

15. Narins RS, Beer K. Liquid injectable silicon: a review of its history, immunology, technical considerations, and potential. Plast Reconstr Surg 2006;118(3S):77S–84S.

16. Truswell WH. Dual-porosity expanded polytetrafluoroethylene soft tissue implant: a new implant for facial soft tissue augmentation. Arch Facial Plast Surg 2002;4:92–7.

17. Verret DJ, Leach JL, Gilmore J. Dual-porosity expanded polytetrafluoroethylene implants for lip, nasolabial groove, and melolabial groove augmentation. Arch Facial Plast Surg 2006;8:423–5.

18. Maas CS, Denton AB. Synthetic soft tissue substitutes 2001. Facial Plast Surg Clin North Am 2001;9:219–27.

19. Constantino PD. Synthetic biomaterials for soft tissue augmentation and replacement in the head and neck. Otolaryngol Clin North Am 1994;27:223–62.

20. Schoenrock LD, Repucci AD. Correction of subcutaneous facial defects using Gore-Tex. Facial Plast Surg Clin North Am 1994;2:373–88.

21. Truswell WH, Mangat DS, Perkins SW, et al. Advanta soft tissue implants—a multicenter review of the first two and one half year's experience. Poster presentation at the American Academy of Facial Plastic and Reconstructive Surgery Fall Meeting. Orlando (FL); 2003.

22. Perkins SW. The corner of the mouth lift and management of the oral commissure grooves. Facial Plast Surg Clin North Am 2007;15(4):471–6.

23. Perkins SW, Sandel HD IV. Anatomic considerations, analysis and the aging process of the perioral region. Facial Plast Surg Clin North Am 2007;15(4):403–7.

24. Waldman SR. The subnasal lift. Facial Plast Surg Clin North Am 2007;15(4):513–6.

REFERENCES: WALDMAN

1. Waldman SR. The subnasal lip lift. Facial Plast Surg Clin North Am 1997;5:65–70.

2. Waldman SR. The subnasal lift. Facial Plast Surg Clin North Am 2007;15(4):513–6.

Mandible Fractures
Discussion and Debate

Oneida Arosarena, MD[a],*, Yadranko Ducic, MD, FRCS(C)[b,c],*,
Travis T. Tollefson, MD, MPH[d],*

KEYWORDS

- Mandible fracture repair • Miniplates • Maxillomandibular fixation • Panel discussion

---

Mandible Fractures Panel Discussion

Oneida Arosarena, Yadro Ducic, and Travis T. Tollefson address questions for discussion and debate:

1. Is rigid fixation essential for the treatment of angle fractures, or is a single plate along the superior border sufficient?

2. Does the presence of teeth in the fracture line (particularly the third molar in angle fractures) contribute to stability of the fixation, or is it a nidus for infection?

3. What is the role of postoperative antibiotics? Are they always necessary?

4. Do you believe that applying MMF is an important part of mandibular fracture repair? If you do not use MMF in all cases, how do you decide which cases require intraoperative and/or postoperative MMF? Do you believe that the techniques/methods of applying MMF make a difference?

5. How do you manage edentulous mandible fractures?

6. *Analysis:* Over the past 5 years, how has your technique or approach changed or what is the most important thing you have learned in dealing with mandible fractures?

Is rigid fixation essential for the treatment of angle fractures, or is a single plate along the superior border sufficient?

AROSARENA

Because of the biomechanics of the mandible, mandibular angle fractures have a high incidence of postsurgical complications. There are currently 2 philosophies espoused by practitioners who use open reduction and internal fixation (ORIF) in the treatment of mandibular angle fractures.

Philosophy 1. The goal of the first group is rigid fixation with 2 miniplates resulting in primary bone union, which necessitates absolute immobility of the fracture fragments according to older Arbeitsgemeinschaft für Osteosynthesefragen–Association for the Study of Internal Fixation guidelines.

---

[a] Department of Otolaryngology–Head and Neck Surgery, Temple University, 3440 North Broad Street, Suite 300, Philadelphia, PA 19128, USA
[b] Department of Otolaryngology–Head and Neck Surgery, University of Texas Southwestern Medical Center, Dallas, TX, USA
[c] Otolaryngology and Facial Plastic Surgery Associates, 923 Pennsylvania Avenue, Suite 100, Fort Worth, TX 76104, USA
[d] Cleft and Craniofacial Program, Otolaryngology–Head and Neck Surgery, Facial Plastic and Reconstructive Surgery, University of California, Davis, 2521 Stockton Boulevard, Suite 7200, Sacramento, CA 95817, USA
* Corresponding authors.
E-mail addresses: oneida@temple.edu; yducic@sbcglobal.net; travis.tollefson@ucdmc.ucdavis.edu

Facial Plast Surg Clin N Am 20 (2012) 347–363
doi:10.1016/j.fsc.2012.05.001
1064-7406/12/$ – see front matter © 2012 Elsevier Inc. All rights reserved.

Philosophy 2. The second group advocates the use of a single miniplate along the ideal line of osteosynthesis as described by Champy. Although this method does not result in rigid fixation, its proponents list benefits of decreased soft-tissue stripping that maintains blood supply to the mandible, the lack of an external incision, and cost savings related to decreased operative time and savings in hardware.[1] Because bite forces do not return to premorbid levels for several weeks after fracture treatment, proponents of the Champy technique argue that absolute rigid fixation may not be necessary for angle fractures.[2]

Several biomechanical studies have demonstrated that the Champy technique has less favorable biomechanical behavior than biplanar plating techniques.[3–7] Two studies revealed that a 3-dimensional plate at the superior border of the mandible resulted in increased stability with torsional loading when compared with other commonly used mandibular angle fixation techniques, effecting biplanar fixation with a single plate.[3,6] However, these studies may represent oversimplified depictions of fractured mandible biomechanics, not taking into account the stabilizing effects of surrounding tissues, particularly muscles.[5,8] Moreover, these models do not take into account the possibility of stress shielding in the healing mandible that could be attributed to rigid fixation.[8,9]

In a prospective, randomized trial of 54 patients with unilateral, isolated mandibular angle fractures, Danda[10] found that the use of 2 noncompression miniplates had no advantage over the use of 1 superior border plate, and that the use of 2 miniplates resulted in scarring at the transcutaneous incision in 18% of patients. However, Danda used 2 weeks of interdental fixation in all patients. Similarly, in a study of 185 patients with isolated unilateral angle fractures, Ellis[1] found no significant difference in treatment outcomes for patients treated with rigid versus nonrigid fixation, although patients treated with rigid fixation in this study had longer operative times and more wound problems. A recent meta-analysis of mandibular angle fixation techniques found lower complication rates with the use of 1 superior border plate compared with the use of 2 plates.[11]

DUCIC

The decision as to which method of fixation is most appropriate will, of course, be determined by the specific type of injury present. There are several options in treating these injuries with respect to fixation modality. Closed reduction is still an option. However, there is a prolonged period of immobilization that may be associated with increased rate of long-term temporomandibular joint problems. Closed reduction is relatively contraindicated in comminuted angle fractures because of the increased risk of complications. Rigid load-bearing plating of angle fractures is needed in comminuted fractures. Compression plating and lag screw fixation is not appropriate in these circumstances, because of the potential for fragmentary telescoping. Studies performed in noncomminuted angle fractures demonstrate a decreased risk of complications with a single superior border monocortical miniplate placed along Champy's ideal line of osteosynthesis, slightly greater complication rate with an inferior border bicortical plate, and the greatest rate of complications with 2 separate plates.[1–5]

TOLLEFSON

In treatment of fractures of craniomaxillofacial skeleton, is it not rigid truth that 2 plates are better than 1? Unfortunately, the relationship of bioengineering concepts to the clinical application of rigid fixation is not as linear as we would expect. Practice patterns in mandible fracture management have steadily evolved over the last century, with surges of major advances from both bioengineering and clinical fields. Ellis[1] recently reported superiority of the single miniplate technique for mandibular angle fractures over either maxillomandibular fixation after closed reduction or 2-plate fixation. He cited fewer complications and shorter operative time. I concur with the application of a single plate at the mandibular oblique line for treatment of angle fractures in the following circumstances:

1. Adequate bone stock is available
2. Comminution or bone defect (eg, gunshot wound) is not present
3. Nonedentulous
4. In the presence of adequate dentition to restore occlusion.

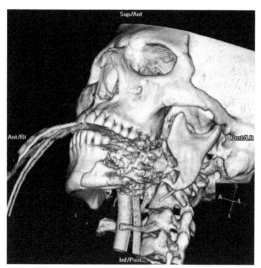

Fig. 1. Mandibular angle fracture open reduction and internal fixation with a single miniplate on the oblique line.

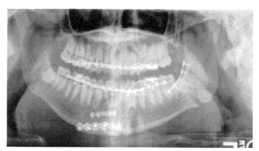

Fig. 3. Following ORIF of both fractures, note persistent lack of reduction at left angle fracture, due to retention of the impacted third molar.

I will briefly introduce the state of the science by reviewing the theories of rigid versus adaptive fixation and the reports of the outcomes of their application.

Without considering the extremes of treatment trends, the contemporary history of mandible fracture treatment paradigms can be simplified into 2 different schools:

1. Treatment patterns restricting function and movement (with external fixation, wires, and load-bearing internal fixation)
2. Shift to near immediate return to function with limited, site-directed internal plate fixation.

The latter incorporates the concept of adaptive osteosynthesis, which has come to be colloquially referred to as the Champy technique in reference

to his expansion on the work of Michelet (Fig. 1).[2] The former, adapted from Association for Osteosynthesis/Association for the Study of Internal Fixation (AO-ASIF) orthopedic management principles of long bone fractures, is supported because of the establishment of rigid fixation for primary bone healing by limiting motion around the fracture (Figs. 1–4).[3]

Conflicting clinical outcomes have been reported using principles of either school, but the fracture site, complexity of the forces applied to the fracture, and independent patient characteristics must be considered. Ellis and Walker[4] reported on angle fracture fixation with 2 miniplates, but later suggested a lower complication rate with a single miniplate.[5] The investigators partially attributed this difference to the additional dissection needed for the second plate. Fox and Kellman[6] contrasted this report with a 2.9% complication rate in 70 angle fractures treated with 2 monocortical miniplates,

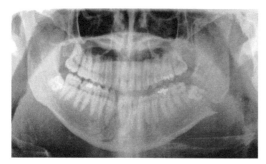

Fig. 2. Preoperative Panorex demonstrating right body and left angle fractures. Note presence of impacted third molar in fracture line.

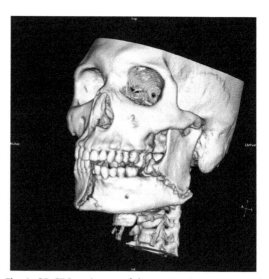

Fig. 4. 3D CT Scan image of demonstrating exposure of the left third molar in the left mandibular angle fracture. A right parasymphyseal fracture is also present.

and also clarified that the 1994 Ellis and Walker study included bicortical application of the inferior border plate. As with any comparative effectiveness research, a direct, randomized prospective study of sufficient power would be ideal, but is unlikely. It is plausible that these contrasting clinical experiences may be clarified by studying outcomes in a multi-institutional database with sufficient collection of fracture details and related secondary factors of bone healing, such as soft-tissue dissection, approaches, technique, and duration of maxillomandibular fixation, and the general patient's general "protoplasm" or health (eg, diabetes, alcoholism, malnutrition, tobacco abuse).

Although the contrasting clinical reports can be difficult to directly compare, I am comfortable with the relative success using either 1 or 2 miniplates on the mandibular angle. I strongly concur with Rudderman and colleagues in that fixation should "provide for a functional construct that can adequately heal while the patient participates in near normal activities."[37] It may seem contradictory to suggest that less fixation is better in some circumstances, but applying functionally stable fixation while allowing dental loads to be applied to the healing mandible may improve bone density, as described by Julius Wolff in 1892 in the law of transformation of bone.[7] The 1-plate technique on the oblique line is my preference for the uncomplicated mandibular angle fracture because it adequately minimizes interfragmentary movement via a limited soft-tissue dissection.

Does the presence of teeth in the fracture line (particularly the third molar in angle fractures) contribute to stability of the fixation, or is it a nidus for infection?

AROSARENA

The prophylactic removal of teeth in the line of fracture was advocated before the widespread use of antibiotics and rigid internal fixation, both of which have significantly reduced the infection rate associated with repair of mandible fractures.[15,16] Retained teeth historically were believed to act as foreign bodies, providing communication between the oral cavity and the periodontal space. The trend over time has been retention of viable teeth in the fracture line.[12,15–19]

Ellis[20] reported a trend toward increased complication rates when molars, particularly the third molar, are involved in the fracture line. However, at least 3 retrospective series demonstrated no difference in outcome of fracture management whether the teeth were routinely extracted or retained, and regardless of whether the fracture was in the anterior or posterior dentition.[17,19,21] The third molar may represent a different situation because it is in a region where debris tends to collect. In a retrospective analysis of 105 mandible fractures associated with incompletely erupted third molars, Rubin and colleagues[22] found a trend toward increased complication rates in cases treated with open reduction when the third molar was retained. Other investigators recommend retention of healthy third molars that do not interfere with fracture reduction, particularly unerupted third molars. They argue that extraction of the third molar reduces contact area in the already thin angular region of the mandible, which may reduce the stability of osteosynthesis and cause micromobility after fixation.[16]

Extraction of viable teeth may induce additional trauma to the adjacent bone and destabilize the fracture. In addition, healthy retained teeth provide a posterior stop, permit proper alignment of the dental arch, and prevent collapsing or telescoping of the fragments. Moreover, a normal coagulum does not always form after tooth extraction, occasionally leading to alveolitis and wound infection.[12,16] According to Spinnato and Alberto,[18] conditions for preserving teeth in the fracture line are antibiotic therapy, strict oral hygiene, radiologic and clinical monitoring for evidence of periapical infection and pulp necrosis, and endodontic therapy for teeth that require treatment. Widely accepted indications for removal of the teeth in the line of fracture include[12,16,18]:

- Significant periodontal disease with gross mobility and periapical pathology
- Partially erupted or erupted third molars with pericoronitis or cystic areas
- Teeth preventing the reduction of fractures
- Teeth with fractured roots
- Teeth with exposed root apices or teeth in which the entire root surface from the apex to the gingival margin is exposed
- Excessive delay from the time of fracture to the time of definitive treatment
- Recurring abscess at the fracture site despite antibiotic therapy.

DUCIC

The presence of a third molar doubles the risk of mandible fracture because of the sheer volume of bone it occupies, effectively diminishing the height of the remaining mandible.[6] There does exist some controversy as to the need for third molar extraction in the setting of mandibular angle fractures. Indications for removal are generally accepted to include the presence of a fractured tooth, a carious tooth, grossly loose or displaced tooth, an impacted third molar that would meet criteria for removal on its own merit, and a tooth preventing adequate fracture reduction. This latter scenario is most often seen with a preoperatively impacted third molar (**Figs. 2 and 3**). If none of these criteria are met then one may consider retaining the tooth based on intraoperative factors. Removing third molars may further diminish the amount of bone remaining across the fracture site and may make the stability of the reduction less stable; this is an intraoperative decision. Several studies support this approach.[7]

TOLLEFSON

Controversy persists over whether to remove a third molar that is in a mandibular angle fracture line. Before the advent of antibiotics, infections in fractures along the tooth-bearing mandible were common. Tooth extraction from the fracture site theoretically decreased bacterial load, but the advent of antibiotics shifted the paradigm.[8] My practice is to retain healthy, erupted molars in mandibular angle fractures with the exception of the indications that I will further describe.

As infection-related complications decreased with the routine use of preoperative and perioperative antibiotics, surgeons began to sort through the effectiveness of different practice patterns: tooth extraction, duration of maxillomandibular fixation, rigid versus adaptive osteosynthesis, and surgical approaches. The debate over third molar extraction in angle fractures excludes an abscessed or severely decayed tooth, which should be extracted in fractures of any area of the mandible. This clinical debate is also partially fueled by the routine practice of preventive extraction of third molar or wisdom teeth, which have had evolving indications and justifications in the oral surgery literature.[9]

Third molars, occupying significant cross-sectional area of the mandibular angle, have been shown to predispose patients to up to 3.8 times the risk of angle fractures than those without third molars.[10–12] Once the fracture is present, some surgeons choose to extract, whereas others retain the third molar. I concur with the theory that extraction of the third molar from a fracture line may destabilize and limit the interfragmentary buttressing required for bone healing (**Fig. 4**).

The literature has support for both extraction and retention of the third molars in angle fractures. The support in the literature for retention is strong. Neal and colleagues[13] and Amaratunga[14] found that removing teeth in the line of a fracture did not change infection rates. The investigators included other tooth-bearing fracture locations in the studies, so we must infer how the angle fractures would behave. Iizuka and Lindqvist[15] went further to suggest that tooth extraction can contribute to postoperative infection. These investigators purport that the tooth extraction may make the fracture site unstable because of diminished bone stock, whereas retaining a tooth may add to stability. In a later study of 121 angle fractures, infection risk was higher after tooth extraction in the fracture line and when compression plate technique was used.[16] The latter practice is now rare.

The support for routine third molar extraction from the fracture line is less convincing. In 1964, Muller[17] supported extraction of teeth with multiple roots from fracture lines. Ellis[18] recently reviewed 400 cases in which third molar extraction from the angle fracture was routine practice. Third molars in the fracture line were present in 85% of the fractures, and 75% of these teeth were removed. Although the difference in infection and

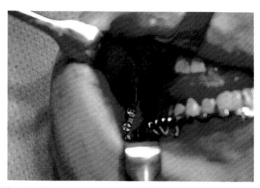

Fig. 5. 3D CT Scan image of demonstrating comminuted fracture of the left left mandibular angle fracture with resulting dental root fractures necessitating extractions.

complication rates failed to reach statistical significance, he concludes that the "difficulty that remains involves determining the appropriate criteria for the removal of teeth in the line of fracture."[18(p865)]

Determining the criteria for extraction remains challenging. My current practice is to retain the third molar in the mandibular fracture line except when the roots are fractured, (Fig. 5) severe dental caries and mobility are present, or in the presence of pericoronitis, abscess, or infection. If extraction of the third molar is required, it can be removed after bone healing, as suggested by Iizuka and Lindquist.[15,16]

What is the role of postoperative antibiotics? Are they always necessary?

AROSARENA

Although the efficacy of perioperative antibiotics in the prevention of orthopedic fracture infections has been established, their use in the treatment of mandibular fractures may not be comparable, due to the increased blood supply to the face but also because mandible fractures involving the tooth-bearing segments of the mandible are, by nature, contaminated wounds. Moreover, the use of postoperative antibiotics in some surgical disciplines has been associated with increased incidence of postoperative infection attributed to the selection of resistant organisms.[23,24] The role of preoperative and intraoperative antibiotics in preventing postoperative infections in the treatment of mandible fractures involving dentate segments is established.[24–26] However, the amount and quality of the existing data on the efficacy of prophylactic postoperative antibiotics in cases of uncomplicated mandible fracture repair is insufficient for formal quantitative synthesis or meta-analysis.[27]

Only 9 randomized controlled trials have addressed the need for postoperative antibiotics after repair of uncomplicated mandible fractures. These trials are limited by being underpowered, and most did not ensure allocation concealment.[26,27] Also, several of the trials utilized various antibiotic regimens and fracture treatment techniques, including closed treatment, within the trial. In a systematic review of 6 of these trials, Andreasen and colleagues[24] determined that antibiotic prophylaxis had no influence on the infection rate when fractures were treated by closed reduction, but significantly reduced the incidence of infection in patients treated with open reduction, because open reduction increases contamination and decreases blood supply to the injured site. None of these studies supported the use of antibiotics beyond the first 48 postoperative hours.[23,24,26]

A randomized, double-blind controlled trial by Abubaker and Rollert[23] studied patients who received postoperative penicillin for 5 days postoperatively in comparison with patients who received placebo. The study demonstrated no benefits to the use of postoperative antibiotics, but included only 30 patients. Other limitations of this study were the exclusion of individuals with immunocompromised states and exclusion of patients who were noncompliant with postoperative medications. Moreover, twice as many patients in the group receiving postoperative antibiotics than those receiving placebo were treated with closed reduction. All of the patients who developed infections were treated with open reduction. The investigators also noted that none of the patients with fractures not involving the angle developed infections.[23]

In a randomized trial including 181 patients, Miles and colleagues[26] noted that of the patients who developed postoperative infections, the use of postoperative antibiotics only delayed the time to presentation with infectious symptoms. In this study the investigators included patients with comminuted fractures, used only open reduction/internal fixation for treatment, and found no benefit to the use of postoperative antibiotics. However, these results should be interpreted with caution because the investigators reported a significant attrition rate (38%), attributed to the patient population (urban, low-income).[26]

In a retrospective study of patients treated for uncomplicated mandible fractures where patients received a variety of antibiotic regimens for varying time periods postoperatively (up to 10 days), Lovato and Wagner[28] found that the use of postoperative antibiotics did not affect postoperative infection rates.

DUCIC

There remains a defined role for perioperative antibiotic therapy in the treatment of mandible fractures. Although postoperative antibiotics are widely as well, studies have not shown them to be necessary or helpful in this patient population.[8,9] In an acutely infected fracture, postoperative antibiotics, covering usual oral pathogens including anaerobes, are generally recommended.[10] In the setting of a chronically infected mandible fracture with osteomyelitis, a prolonged course of antibiotic therapy that may extend as long as 6 weeks is recommended.

TOLLEFSON

To answer this question, we must clarify the current practice trends that differ by surgeon, geography, specialty, and even individual case. An infected mandible fracture site demonstrating erythema, purulence, cutaneous fistula, or malunion/nonunion is a clear indication for antibiotics. However, we must consider the utility of the postoperative antibiotic course, especially involving fractures of the dentoalveolar segments caused by the inherent oral bacterial contamination.[20,22,23]

Antibiotic usage can by administered at different time points in treatment, including time of diagnosis, immediately preoperatively, for a 24-hour postoperative period, and as extended postoperative treatment (7–10 days). The doctrine of using of preoperative antibiotics given 1 hour before surgery comes from the general surgery literature.[26,27] Antibiotic prophylaxis for orthopedic fractures are often discontinued within 24 hours postoperatively.[24,25] The value of preoperative antibiotics when the fracture involves a tooth-bearing segment is strongly supported.[23,29] The study by Zallen and Curry[22] compared exposure to either no antibiotics or any antibiotics in open and closed reduction treatments of a variety of mandible fracture locations, and they reported a strikingly higher infection rate in the nonantibiotic groups (50.33%) compared with receiving any antibiotic (6.25%). None of these studies provided specific information on the value of postoperative antibiotics.

Abubaker and Rollert[21] designed a prospective, double-blind, clinical study to investigate the effect of postoperative antibiotics. All patients received penicillin G perioperatively and for 12 hours postoperatively while the second arm received additional penicillin VK orally for 5 days, and the control group received placebo. The investigators found that "postoperative oral antibiotics in uncomplicated fractures of the mandible had no benefit in reducing the incidence of infection."[21] These findings concur with those of Furr and colleagues,[19] who also noted no difference in those cases that had delayed treatment. However, alcohol and tobacco abuse was associated with increased complications such as abscess, infection, nonunion/malunion, and hardware exposure. It may be that algorithms for antibiotic use will need to consider these as well as other patient-specific risk factors.

This difficult clinical question is fueled by conflicting evidence from mostly experiential data that may not be generalizable. Kyzas[28] recently called for large, randomized controlled trials after performing a systematic review of 31 studies, which included 9 randomized control trials and more than 5000 cases. This analysis failed to answer the question of the effectiveness of antibiotic use in mandible fractures. Lovato and Wagner[29] reported no difference in infection rate when patients with mandible fractures were treated only perioperatively (13.33%) or for up to 7 days postoperatively (10.67%). Of note, this case-control study of 150 cases included closed reduction cases, which may have risks different to those of ORIF.

In reviewing the available literature, the retrospective approach has many limitations, not the least of which include a lack of consistent data collection. The ideal study would include the following factors:

1. Timing of surgery after injury
2. Site of mandible fractures (eg, decreased infection risk in non–tooth-bearing condylar and ramus fractures)
3. Type and dosage of antibiotic
4. Timing of antibiotic administration including presurgical, intraoperative, and postoperative
5. Duration of antibiotic course
6. Surgical approach (external or intraoral)
7. Fixation technique (ORIF or closed reduction with maxillomandibular fixation).

Although multi-institutional, randomized control trials would be valuable for antibiotics in facial fracture treatment, the study design is often deemed impractical or unfeasible. The best alternative comparative study would need to account for the differences in patient demographics, health status, tobacco and alcohol use, and dental health.

My preference for antibiotic use will continue to include pre-, peri-, and postoperative as we await potential definitive, future studies that may include more of the 7 factors listed above. My protocol includes giving antibiotics at the time of presentation until the repair, relaying on oral clindamycin or penicillin or intravenous clindamycin or cefazolin. The dosage given an hour before surgery is given intravenously and then repeated until conversion to the oral equivalent, which, along with 0.1% chlorhexidine rinses, is continued for 7 days.

There seems to be a recent trend toward repairing mandible fractures without applying MMF. Do you believe that applying MMF is an important part of mandibular fracture repair? If you do not use MMF in all cases, how do you decide which cases require intraoperative and/or postoperative MMF? Do you believe that the techniques/methods of applying MMF make a difference?

AROSARENA

While there is a trend toward repairing mandible fractures without applying maxillomandibular fixation (MMF), I believe that MMF is important in dentulous patients, to establish normal occlusion in fractures involving the dental arch. In cases of fractures distal to the dental arch, when there is postoperative malocclusion due to masticator muscle dysfunction or soft-tissue swelling, I also use elastic interdental fixation to guide the patient into normal occlusion. Interdental fixation, obviously, is also used for subcondylar or condylar fractures treated with closed reduction. I do not typically use MMF if the mandible is edentulous or has so few teeth that occlusion cannot be established; in these cases I believe that dentures can be adjusted to address postoperative malocclusion, if present. Although I have used MMF screws in the past, my preference is the traditional arch bars with circumdental wiring. I have found difficulty with maintaining stable occlusion with MMF screws, and they cannot be used for postoperative elastic interdental fixation if necessary. Moreover, arch bars are effective at reducing and stabilizing comminuted fractures involving the alveolar ridge.

DUCIC

Maintaining or reestablishing proper occlusion is one of the most important goals in mandible fracture repair. Multiple methods exist for this purpose. Intraoperative MMF such as with MMF screws is a rapid and effective method we use in 2 scenarios:

1. Where the patient's dentition is too poor or inadequate to accept proper arch bar fixation.

2. Where there is no anticipation of needing postoperative guiding elastics.

In situations where there may be a need for postoperative guiding elastics such as subcondylar fractures, comminuted fractures, or multiple fractures of the mandible, it would be the unusual patient who would not benefit from traditional MMF with arch bars. This approach remains the gold standard.

TOLLEFSON

I choose to use MMF for mandible fracture stabilization in:

1. Nearly all isolated condyle, ramus, angle, and body fractures
2. Those patients with 2 or more fracture sites (**Fig. 6**).

In patients with adequate dentition I prefer an open approach for fracture reduction, which affords intraoperative visualization of the fracture segments while reproducing the dental occlusion (based on wear facets and classic definitions). MMF is maintained to stabilize occlusion during ORIF. I prefer to leave the arch bars in place and apply guiding elastics for up to 4 weeks.

There are 3 broad categories in which I will defer MMF: isolated anterior fractures; pediatric cases; and when absent, diseased dentition precludes its use. I choose Ernst ligatures in those cases where only one fracture in the anterior mandible (symphyseal/parasymphyseal fractures) is present, and then remove them after ORIF. Similarly in pediatric cases, ligatures or MMF will be removed after ORIF except when addressing condylar fractures with functional adaptation.

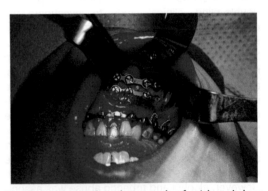

Fig. 6. Intraoperative photograph of erich arch bars and two miniplates used for fixation of a right mandibular parasymphyseal fracture. Maxillomandibular fixation was used due to a concomitant left mandibular angle fracture. Guiding elastics were used post-operatively.

Although some surgeons support the use of intermaxillary fixation (IMF) screws for fixation, I rarely use this option.[30] The screws can become mobile in the maxillary segment and are not intended to allow long-term fixation or guiding elastic capability. The risk of tooth-bud injury with IMF screw placement makes circumdental wires my preference in pediatric cases.

How do you manage edentulous mandible fractures?

AROSARENA

The edentulous mandible is typically atrophic. I usually manage angle and body fractures in the edentulous mandible with a single 2.4-mm locking reconstruction plate for stability. I treat unilateral condylar and subcondylar fractures in the edentulous mandible conservatively (soft mechanical diet or liquid diet). In the few instances when I have treated edentulous patients with bilateral condylar and subcondylar fractures, I have approached these through the parotid, with care being taken to dissect and preserve the facial nerve, and have rigidly fixed the fractures with 2.0-mm plates (one at each fracture site).

DUCIC

This would depend mostly on the patient's mandible height across the fracture line. If the height is at least 20 mm, it is treated as for any mandible fracture in the nonedentulous patient. If the height is between 10 and 19 mm, we will use rigid fixation with iliac or other bone graft packed around the fracture site. If the height is less than 10 mm then a weight-bearing fixation method with a large locking screw plate and major bone grafting is often required. Subperiosteal versus supraperiosteal plate placement seems not to be important when the studies are compared in this regard. Controlling underlying medical problems that are often seen in the elderly edentulous patient population is important, as these may also affect healing.

TOLLEFSON

I believe that the use of soft diet and conservative observation for edentulous mandible fractures should only be used in the frailest patients, who would not tolerate general anesthesia. Otherwise, the premorbid jaw position can be estimated by using the patient's dentures, but these nearly always need to be altered or refabricated after the large 2.4-mm mandibular locking plate is applied to the fracture(s) through an external approach. In a rare case where complex maxillary fractures and an edentulous mandible fracture are present, I will complete MMF by modifying the patient's dentures with drill holes, or our dentist will fabricate a Gunning splint. These cases often receive a tracheotomy, obviating the urge to remove the MMF in the immediate postoperative period. I advocate an external approach to complete the load-bearing ORIF of edentulous mandible fractures. In cases with 2 fractures, I choose a large plate that extends through both fractures with 3 or more screws on each side of the fracture. In the primary setting, if the fracture segments involve "pencil-thin" or osteoporotic bone, I prefer the iliac crest as the cancellous bone graft harvest site.

Analysis: Over the past 5 years, how has your technique or approach changed or what is the most important thing you have learned in dealing with mandible fractures?

AROSARENA

Contemplation on mandibular angle fractures
The method of fixation of mandibular angle fractures that I have used and that has resulted in the fewest postoperative complications in terms of infection is a transcutaneous approach with a non-compression, 6-hole miniplate placed along the inferior border and secured with bicortical screws, in conjunction with a 4-hole tension band secured with monocortical screws so as not to injure the inferior alveolar nerve (**Fig. 7**). I believe that this approach minimizes the exposure of the bone to the contaminated oral cavity, and because a drain is placed, the risk of hematoma is minimized. However, because I have had patients develop hypertrophic scarring and transient facial nerve

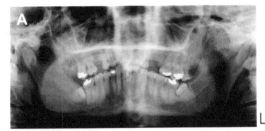
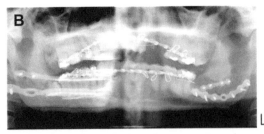

Fig. 7. Orthopantograms of a 46-year-old man with an isolated left mandibular angle fracture. (*A*) Preoperative orthopantogram. (*B*) Postoperative orthopantogram showing fracture fixation with a 7-hole miniplate placed near the inferior border with a 4-hole tension band. The approach was transcutaneous.

injury with this approach, my current preference is a biplanar technique with a miniplate placed at the internal oblique line with monocortical screws, and a second miniplate placed just below this on the buccal cortex with bicortical screws using a transbuccal trocar (**Fig. 8**). Although this has resulted in noticeable scars in a few patients, I believe that this technique affords enough stability to overcome distractive and torsional forces, especially if the third molar has to be removed because it is carious, has broken roots, or is impeding fracture reduction. Removal of the third molar significantly

reduces the stability of the mandible in the angle region, and I do not believe that a single miniplate can restore adequate stability for uncomplicated bone healing when the third molar has to be extracted.[9,12] I have used the Champy technique in instances when the fracture was minimally displaced and the third molar did not have to be extracted, and I have also used a single miniplate along the buccal cortex (**Fig. 9**). Like other investigators, I have not noted an increase in complications whether 1 miniplate or 2 miniplates were used for angle fracture management.[7,10,13,14]

Contemplation on teeth in the fracture line

Despite the trend in the literature to retain teeth in the line of fracture, I find that the criteria for preserving teeth (strict oral hygiene, radiologic and clinical monitoring) often cannot be met in the patient

population I serve at an inner-city, tertiary care, academic medical center. Moreover, many of my patients have no access to endodontic therapy given their uninsured status. Thus, the viability of

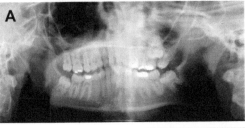
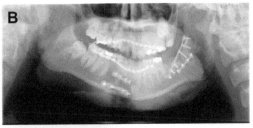
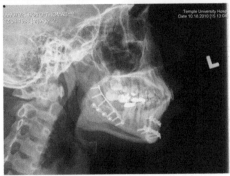

Fig. 8. Radiographs of a 19-year-old man with a left mandibular angle and right parasymphyseal mandibular fractures. (*A*) Preoperative orthopantogram. (*B*) Postoperative orthopantogram demonstrating placement of a miniplate along the oblique line with a second plate placed just below this along the buccal cortex. (*C*) Lateral mandibular radiograph taken 2 years after the initial injury, demonstrating healing of the fracture.

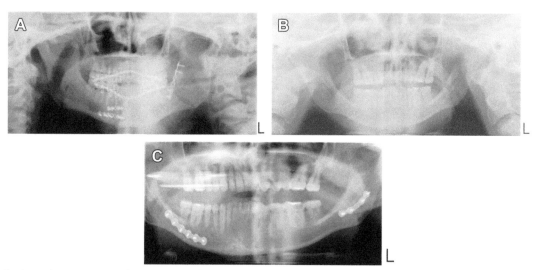

Fig. 9. Orthopantograms demonstrating fixation of mandibular angle fractures with a single miniplate. (*A*) Postoperative orthopantogram demonstrating fixation of a left mandibular angle fracture with the Champy technique in a 33-year-old man. (*B*) Preoperative orthopantogram of a 22-year-old man with left angle and right body mandibular fractures. (*C*) Orthopantogram of patient in *B* taken 1 month after fixation of angle fracture with a single plate along the buccal cortex.

the tooth is only one consideration in my decisions to preserve or extract teeth in the line of fracture. In fact, I believe that a tendency on my part to be too conservative with tooth extraction has resulted in some unnecessary complications. At least 2 cases of postsurgical infection resulted from my decision to preserve viable-appearing, stable teeth despite the roots being partially exposed (**Figs. 10** and **11**). I am now more aggressive with removal of teeth with exposed roots.

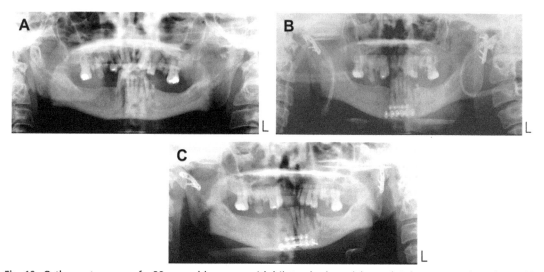

Fig. 10. Orthopantograms of a 38-year-old woman with bilateral subcondylar and right parasymphyseal mandibular fractures. (*A*) Preoperative orthopantogram. (*B*) Postoperative orthopantogram demonstrating ORIF of fractures. The subcondylar fractures were repaired via transparotid approaches given the patient's poor dentition. During repair of the right parasymphyseal fracture, the decision was made to retain the tooth mesial to the fracture because it seemed stable and healthy. (*C*) Orthopantogram taken 2 weeks after fracture repair when patient returned with infection at the fracture line. The nonunion healed with removal of the tooth at the fracture line and conservative treatment with antibiotics.

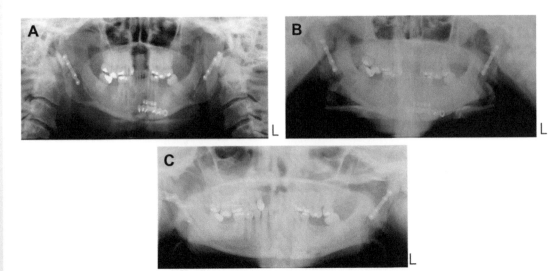

Fig. 11. Orthopantograms of a 51-year-old man with bilateral subcondylar and left parasymphyseal mandibular fractures. (*A*) Immediate postoperative orthopantogram demonstrating good reduction of fractures. The subcondylar fractures were repaired via a transparotid approach. (*B*) The patient presented with pain and granulation tissue at the site of the parasymphyseal fracture 2 months after repair, and this orthopantogram demonstrated nonunion of that fracture. (*C*) Orthopantogram taken 7 months after initial repair. In the interim between this radiograph and that in *B*, the patient was taken to the operating room where he was found to have partial union of the lingual cortex of the mandible at the parasymphyseal fracture site. The decision was made to remove the hardware and do nothing more.

Contemplation on postoperative antibiotics

Orthognathic surgery is analogous to the treatment of mandible fractures in that osteotomies are made within the same contaminated oral cavity environment, although the infection rates with orthognathic surgery are considerably lower than those with mandible fracture treatment, and most studies have not shown prophylactic antibiotics to be preventive in orthognathic surgery.[24] This finding indicates that factors beside the contaminated field are operative in the pathogenesis of infections associated with mandible fractures. It is impossible for studies to control for all of these factors, which include, but are not limited to: (1) delay in treatment, (2) periodontal disease, (3) other comorbidities, (4) imperfect social situation, (5) patient noncompliance, and (6) teeth in the line of fracture. In my practice, most patients with facial trauma present with several of the aforementioned factors, so the use of prophylactic postoperative antibiotics must be individualized.

Delay in treatment It is not unusual to have patients present for initial evaluation several weeks after suffering a mandible fracture. In other instances, patients with multiple injuries, particularly those with intracranial hemorrhages, cervical spine fractures, and other central nervous system insults, may have definitive treatment of facial fractures delayed several days until the patient's other conditions stabilize. In their study of 101 patients with facial fractures, Chole and Yee[25] did not find that delay of treatment affected infection rate, with or without the use of perioperative antibiotics. However, the average delay of treatment for patients in this study was less than 2 days, and the investigators conceded that the protocol was not designed to study the effects of treatment delay, so that these data were retrospective in nature.[25] Fox and Kellman[29] also noted that delay in treatment did not statistically increase the complication rate in their study, but did not specify the average delay period in their series. In a study where approximately 76% of patients presented after 3 days for treatment of facial fractures, and 36% presented between 3 and 10 days, Abiose[30] reported a 56% infection rate despite the use of perioperative antibiotics. The two cases of osteomyelitis of the mandible resulting from fractures that I treated occurred in patients who presented late for treatment, one of whom presented with an abscess. I routinely provide a 5-day course of postoperative antibiotics for patients with a treatment delay of several days.

Periodontal disease and other comorbidities Periodontal disease predisposes to postoperative infections in the treatment of mandible fractures, and is associated with poor dental hygiene.[18] Other comorbidities such as diabetes, human immuno-deficiency virus (HIV) disease, malnutrition, and substance abuse are also associated with infections, the latter being closely linked to patient noncompliance. In their study, in which patients were recruited from a population similar to the one I serve, Miles and colleagues[26] found that only 3 of the 22 patients who developed infections after open treatment of mandible fractures had past medical histories (HIV disease, hepatitis C infection

with cirrhosis) that may have predisposed to infection. Again, these results may be skewed by the high attrition rate in this study. However, they did demonstrate that infections were more prevalent in patients with combined alcohol and tobacco use.[26] Similarly, Lovato and Wagner[28] found that the incidence of infection was higher in patients with a history of drug use. I prescribe postoperative antibiotics for patients with periodontal disease and other comorbidities.

Social situation Compliance with postoperative instructions, including the use of oral rinses, and dental hygiene is often difficult for populations that are transient, homeless, and indigent. I had one homeless patient who was discharged without antibiotics return 3 weeks later with a deep neck infection arising from his parasymphyseal fracture

site. After successful treatment of the infection, the fracture went on to heal, although the patient did not return for follow-up after his second hospitalization until a year later because his arch bars were becoming a nuisance to him. As these are patients who also tend to have significant comorbidities, I discharge them with a short course of antibiotics.

Teeth in the line of fracture One of the stated conditions for maintenance of teeth in the line of fracture is antibiotic prophylaxis.[18] Before the antibiotic era routine extraction of teeth in the line of fracture was advocated, because of the risks of osteomyelitis and nonunion. Although teeth in the

line of fracture may not increase these risks in patients with good dentition and dental hygiene, I am inclined to give antibiotic prophylaxis in patients with poor dentition and/or poor dental hygiene for the stated reasons.

DUCIC

Over the past few years I have transitioned to less and less need for MMF. There is a tendency to a greater use of intraoperative arch bars or MMF screws with removal at the completion of the procedure. In addition, very few patients require MMF postoperatively and most are mobilized as

soon as possible. Also, greater reliance on 2 monocortical miniplates for noncomminuted body and symphyseal fractures and less reliance on more rigid techniques has been associated with increased ease of fixation and favorable postoperative outcomes.

TOLLEFSON

As surgeons shift toward a more objective, evidence-based analysis of surgical outcomes, the expert opinion will inherently affect practice trends to a diminishing degree. The experienced surgeon's opinion will still be valuable, as experiential learning is especially important in the less prevalent surgical treatments. However, the opinion will be shaped by research that draws from evidence-based medicine, emphasizing systematic reviews and prospective cohort studies over case reports and small retrospective reviews.[31,32] This process, similar to Epstein's description of observational analysis, will be "established by comparisons, by shifting shades of difference, turned over and teased out".[33]

My practice habits in mandible fracture management have changed in, at least, the following trends:

1. Increased use of functionally stable fixation[37]
2. Use of an envelope vestibular incision for angle fractures when the third molar is extracted

3. Approach and fixation in uncomplicated angle fractures
4. Immediate use of guiding elastics
5. Use of resorbable plates for pediatric cases.

The first 3 listed are thoroughly discussed in the discussion topics 1 and 2. As surgeons moved away from inferior border compression plates, the use of adaptive osteosynthesis has gained attention. My experience in using one miniplate on the oblique line in angle fractures is consistent with the other reports that support the theory of lines of osteosynthesis.[34–36] If an angle fracture has significant comminution, then traditional plating through an external approach is my preference. Five years ago, I used a transoral/transbuccal approach to place 2 plates on the lateral surface of angle with bicortical screws in the inferior border.

From exposure to oral surgery colleagues in the AO-ASIF, I began using an envelope vestibular incision for transoral angle fracture repair in cases that necessitated the removal of a loose or de-cayed third molar in the fracture line. Using this incision, the gingiva is lifted directly from the molars and then extends posteriorly in the standard vestibular incision. This approach has the benefit of affording mucosal closure over the socket. In general, I attempt to limit periosteal dissection in uncomplicated fractures and will use 2 monocortical miniplates in nondisplaced, parasymphyseal fractures, instead of a larger inferior border, bicortical application.

I still prefer Erich arch bar application over 4-screw MMF screw systems, but have shifted away from wire fixation at the end of surgery. Guiding elastics are used immediately postoperatively and continued for 2 to 6 weeks depending on the patient's malocclusion potential. This practice theoretically promotes bone growth by applying an early load to the mandible during healing.[37] Lastly, in a limited number of pediatric mandible cases, I have found the absorbable plating systems to have both benefits and limitations. The absorbable plates certainly preclude the need for reoperation to remove titanium hardware in a growing mandible. However, if MMF is still used then the child needs a second anesthesia to remove the arch bars as well. Rigid fixation for pediatric cases ideally will be strong enough to obviate postoperative MMF, while absorbing rapidly enough to limit the time-limited edema from the implant.

Mandible fracture management trends have shifted from immobilization, to wire osteosynthesis, to ORIF with large, load-bearing plates. Current recommendations for some fractures support periosteal dissection, less plating, and early return to function. Discussions and collaborative studies between surgeons will help guide us to drive innovative practices at a pace that allows evolution, but with cautious investigation, as the bar continues to be set higher within facial fracture management.

REFERENCES: AROSARENA

1. Ellis E. A prospective study of 3 treatment methods for isolated fractures of the mandibular angle. J Oral Maxillofac Surg 2010;68:2743–54.
2. Ellis E. Treatment methods for fractures of the mandibular angle. Int J Oral Maxillofac Surg 1999;28:243–52.
3. Alkan A, Çelebi N, Özden B, et al. Biomechanical comparison of different plating techniques in repair of mandibular angle fractures. Oral Surg Oral Med Oral Pathol Oral Radiol Endod 2007;104:752–6.
4. Choi BH, Kim KN, Kang HS. Clinical and in vitro evaluation of mandibular angle fracture fixation with the two-miniplate system. Oral Surg Oral Med Oral Pathol Oral Radiol Endod 1995;79:692–5.
5. Fedok FG, van Kooten DW, deJoseph LM, et al. Plating techniques and plate orientation in repair of mandibular angle fractures: an in vitro study. Laryngoscope 1998;108:1218–24.
6. Kalfarentzos EF, Deligianni D, Mitros G, et al. Biomechanical evaluation of plating techniques for fixing mandibular angle fractures: the introduction of a new 3D plate approach. Oral Maxillofac Surg 2009;13:139–44.
7. Schierle HP, Schmelzeisen R, Rahn B, et al. One- or two-plate fixation of mandibular angle fractures? J Craniomaxillofac Surg 1997;25:162–8.
8. Rudderman RH, Mullen RL, Phillips JH. The biophysics of mandibular fractures: an evolution toward understanding. Plast Reconstr Surg 2008;121:596–607.
9. Levy FE, Smith RW, Odland RM, et al. Monocortical miniplate fixation of mandibular angle fractures. Arch Otolaryngol Head Neck Surg 1991;117:149–54.
10. Danda AK. Comparison of a single noncompression miniplate versus 2 noncompression miniplates in the treatment of mandibular angle fractures: a prospective, randomized clinical trial. J Oral Maxillofac Surg 2010;68:1565–7.
11. Regev E, Shiff JS, Kiss A, et al. Internal fixation of mandibular angle fractures: a meta-analysis. Plast Reconstr Surg 2010;125:1753–60.
12. Shetty V, Freymiller E. Teeth in the line of fracture: a review. J Oral Maxillofac Surg 1989;47:1303–6.
13. Seemann R, Schicho K, Wutzl A, et al. Complication rates in the operative treatment of mandibular angle fractures: a 10-year retrospective. J Oral Maxillofac Surg 2010;68:647–50.
14. Siddiqui A, Markose G, Moos KF, et al. One miniplate versus two in the management of mandibular angle fractures: a prospective randomised study. Br J Oral Maxillofac Surg 2007;45:223–5.
15. Chambers IG, Scully C. Mandibular fractures in India during the Second World War (1944 and 1945): analysis of the Snawdon series. Br J Oral Maxillofac Surg 1987;25:357–69.
16. Gerbino G, Tarello F, Fasolis M, et al. Rigid fixation with teeth in the line of mandibular fractures. Int J Oral Maxillofac Surg 1997;26:182–6.
17. De Amaratunga NA. The effect of teeth in the line of mandibular fractures on healing. J Oral Maxillofac Surg 1987;45:312–4.

18. Spinnato G, Alberto PL. Teeth in the line of mandibular fractures. Atlas Oral Maxillofac Surg Clin North Am 2009;17:15–8.

19. Thaller SR, Mabourakh S. Teeth located in the line of mandibular fracture. J Craniofac Surg 1994;5:16–9.

20. Ellis E. Outcomes of patients with teeth in the line of mandibular angle fractures treated with stable internal fixation. J Oral Maxillofac Surg 2002;60: 863–5.

21. Chuong R, Donoff RB, Guralnick WC. A retrospective analysis of 327 mandibular fractures. J Oral Maxillofac Surg 1983;41:305–9.

22. Rubin MM, Koll TJ, Sadoff RS. Morbidity associated with incompletely erupted third molars in the line of mandibular fractures. J Oral Maxillofac Surg 1990; 48:1045–7.

23. Abubaker AO, Rollert MK. Postoperative antibiotic prophylaxis in mandibular fractures: a preliminary randomized, double-blind, and placebo-controlled clinical study. J Oral Maxillofac Surg 2001;59: 1415–9.

24. Andreasen JO, Jensen SS, Schwartz O, et al. A systematic review of prophylactic antibiotics in the surgical treatment of maxillofacial fractures. J Oral Maxillofac Surg 2006;64:1664–8.

25. Chole RA, Yee J. Antibiotic prophylaxis for facial fractures: a prospective, randomized clinical trial. Arch Otolaryngol Head Neck Surg 1987;113:1055–7.

26. Miles BA, Potter JK, Ellis E. The efficacy of postoperative antibiotic regimens in the open treatment of mandibular fractures: a prospective randomized trial. J Oral Maxillofac Surg 2006;64:576–82.

27. Kyzas PA. Use of antibiotics in the treatment of mandible fractures: a systematic review. J Oral Maxillofac Surg 2011;69:1129–45.

28. Lovato C, Wagner JD. Infection rates following perioperative prophylactic antibiotics versus postoperative extended regimen prophylactic antibiotics in surgical management of mandibular fractures. J Oral Maxillofac Surg 2009;67:827–32.

29. Fox AJ, Kellman RM. Mandibular angle fractures: two-miniplate fixation and complications. Arch Facial Plast Surg 2003;5:464–9.

30. Abiose BO. Maxillofacial skeleton injuries in the western states of Nigeria. Br J Oral Maxillofac Surg 1986;24:31–9.

REFERENCES: DUCIC

1. Danda AK. Comparison of a single noncompression miniplate versus 2 noncompression miniplates in the treatment of mandibular angle fractures: a prospective, randomized clinical trial. J Oral Maxillofac Surg 2010;68(7):1565–7.

2. Ellis E. Management of fractures through the angle of the mandible. Oral Maxillofac Surg Clin North Am 2009;21(2):163–74.

3. Ellis E. Treatment methods for fractures of the mandibular angle. Int J Oral Maxillofac Surg 1999; 28(4):243–52.

4. Ellis E 3rd, Walker LR. Treatment of mandibular angle fractures using one noncompression miniplate. J Oral Maxillofac Surg 1996;54(7):864–71 [discussion: 871–2].

5. Fox AJ, Kellman RM. Mandibular angle fractures: two-miniplate fixation and complications. Arch Facial Plast Surg 2003;5(6):464–9.

6. Bezerra TP, Studart-Soares EC, Pita-Neto IC, et al. Do third molars weaken the mandibular angle? Med Oral Patol Oral Cir Bucal 2011;16(5):e657–63.

7. Halmos DR, Ellis E 3rd, Dodson TB. Mandibular third molars and angle fractures. J Oral Maxillofac Surg 2004;62(9):1076–81.

8. Kyzas PA. Use of antibiotics in the treatment of mandible fractures: a systematic review. J Oral Maxillofac Surg 2011;69(4):1129–45.

9. Miles BA, Potter JK, Ellis E 3rd. The efficacy of postoperative antibiotic regimens in the open treatment of mandibular fractures: a prospective randomized trial. J Oral Maxillofac Surg 2006;64(4):576–82.

10. Mehra P, Van Heukelom E, Cottrell DA. Rigid internal fixation of infected mandibular fractures. J Oral Maxillofac Surg 2009;67(5):1046–51.

REFERENCES: TOLLEFSON: RIGID FIXATION

1. Ellis E 3rd. A prospective study of 3 treatment methods for isolated fractures of the mandibular angle. J Oral Maxillofac Surg 2010;68(11):2743–54.

2. Champy M, Lodde JP, Schmitt R, et al. Mandibular osteosynthesis by miniature screwed plates via a buccal approach. J Maxillofac Surg 1978;6:14–21.

3. Spiessl B. Rigid internal fixation of fractures of the lower jaw. Reconstr Surg Traumatol 1972;13:124–40.

4. Ellis E, Walker L. Treatment of mandibular angle fractures using two noncompression miniplates. J Oral Maxillofac Surg 1994;52:1032–6.

5. Ellis E, Walker L. Treatment of mandibular angle fractures using one noncompression miniplate. J Oral Maxillofac Surg 1996;54:864–71.

6. Fox AJ, Kellman RM. Mandibular angle fractures two-miniplate fixation and complications. Arch Facial Plast Surg 2003;5:464–9.

7. Wolff J. The law of bone remodeling. Berlin, Heidelberg, New York: Springer; 1986 (translation of the German 1892 edition).

REFERENCES: TOLLEFSON: PRESENCE OF HEALTHY TEETH

8. Ellis E 3rd. Management of fractures through the angle of the mandible. Oral Maxillofac Surg Clin North Am 2009;21(2):163–74.
9. Bishara SE. Third molars: a dilemma! or is it? Am J Orthod Dentofacial Orthop 1999;115:628–33.
10. Sinn DP, Ghali GE. Morbidity associated with incompletely erupted third molars in the line of mandibular fractures. J Oral Maxillofac Surg 1990;48(10):1048.
11. Subhashraj K. A study on the impact of mandibular third molars on angle fractures. J Oral Maxillofac Surg 2009;67(5):968–72.
12. Tevepaugh DB, Dodson TB. Are mandibular third molars a risk factor for angle fractures? A retrospective cohort study. J Oral Maxillofac Surg 1995;53(6):646–9.
13. Neal DC, Wagner WF, Alpert B. Morbidity associated with teeth in the line of mandibular fractures. J Oral Surg 1978;36(11):859–62.
14. Amaratunga NA. The effect of teeth in the line of mandibular fractures on healing. J Oral Maxillofac Surg 1987;45(4):312–4.
15. Iizuka T, Lindqvist C, Hallikainen D, et al. Infection after rigid internal fixation of mandibular fractures. A clinical and radiological study. J Oral Maxillofac Surg 1991;49:585.
16. Iizuka T, Lindqvist C. Rigid internal fixation of fractures in the angular region of the mandible: an analysis of factors contributing to different complications. Plast Reconstr Surg 1993;91:265–71.
17. Muller W. Zur Frage des Versuchs der Erhaltung der im Bruchspaltstehenden Zähne unter antibiotischem Schutz. Dtsch Zahn Mund Kieferheilk 1964;41:360.
18. Ellis E. Outcomes of patients with teeth in the line of mandibular angle fractures treated with stable internal fixation. J Oral Maxillofac Surg 2002;60:863–5.

REFERENCES: TOLLEFSON: POSTOPERATIVE ANTIBIOTICS

19. Furr AM, Schweinfurth J, May WL. Factors associated with long-term complications after repair of mandibular fractures. Laryngoscope 2006;116:427–30.
20. Miles B, Potter J, Ellis E. The efficacy of postoperative antibiotic regimens in the open treatment of mandibular fractures: a prospective randomized trial. J Oral Maxillofac Surg 2006;64(4):576–82.
21. Abubaker AO, Rollert MK. Postoperative antibiotic prophylaxis in mandibular fractures: a preliminary randomized, double-blind, and placebo-controlled clinical study. J Oral Maxillofac Surg 2001;59(12):1415–9.
22. Zallen RD, Curry J. A study of antibiotic usage in compound mandibular fractures. J Oral Surg 1975; 33:431–4.
23. Greenberg RN, James RB, Marier RL, et al. Microbiologic and antibiotic aspects of infections in the oral and maxillofacial region. J Oral Surg 1979;37:873–84.
24. Page CP, Bohnen JM, Fletcher JR, et al. Antimicrobial prophylaxis for surgical wounds. Guidelines for clinical care. Arch Surg 1993;128:79–88.
25. Nelson CL, Green TG, Porter RA, et al. One day versus seven days of preventative antibiotic therapy in orthopaedic surgery. Clin Orthop 1983; 176:258–63.
26. Burke JF. The effective period of preventative antibiotic action in experimental incisions and dermal lesions. Surgery 1961;50:161–8.
27. Classen DC, Evans RS, Pestotnik SL, et al. The timing of prophylactic administration of antibiotics and the risk of surgical wound infection. N Engl J Med 1992;326:281–6.
28. Kyzas PA. Use of antibiotics in the treatment of mandible fractures: a systematic review. J Oral Maxillofac Surg 2011;69(4):1129–45.
29. Lovato C, Wagner JD. Infection rates following perioperative prophylactic antibiotics versus postoperative extended regimen prophylactic antibiotics in surgical management of mandibular fractures. J Oral Maxillofac Surg 2009;67(4):827–32.

REFERENCE: TOLLEFSON: MMF

30. Ansari K, Hamlar D, Ho V, et al. A comparison of anterior vs posterior isolated mandible fractures treated with intermaxillary fixation screws. Arch Facial Plast Surg 2011;13(4):266–70.

REFERENCES: TOLLEFSON: ANALYSIS OF TECHNIQUE

31. Evidence-Based Medicine Working Group. Evidence-based medicine: a new approach to teaching the practice of medicine. JAMA 1992; 268(17):2420–5.
32. Chung KC, Swanson JA, Schmitz D, et al. Introducing evidence based medicine to plastics and reconstructive surgery. Plast Reconstr Surg 2009; 123(4):1385–9.
33. Epstein J. Friendship: an expose. New York: Houghton Migglin; 2006. p. 11.
34. Champy M, Lodde JP, Schmitt R, et al. Mandibular osteosynthesis by miniature screwed plates

via a buccal approach. J Maxillofac Surg 1978;6: 14–21.

35. Ellis E, Walker L. Treatment of mandibular angle fractures using one noncompression miniplate. J Oral Maxillofac Surg 1996;54: 864–71.

36. Ellis E 3rd. A prospective study of 3 treatment methods for isolated fractures of the mandibular angle. J Oral Maxillofac Surg 2010;68(11):2743–54.

37. Rudderman RH, Mullen RL, Phillips JH. The biophysics of mandibular fractures: an evolution toward understanding. Plast Reconstr Surg 2008;121:596.

Subcondylar Fractures

Edward Ellis III, DDS, MS[a],*, Robert M. Kellman, MD[c],*,
Emre Vural, MD[b],*

KEYWORDS

- Subcondylar fracture • Mandible fracture • Facial fracture • Surgical techniques
- Open surgical technique • Closed surgical technique • Mandible maxilla

---

Subcondylar Fractures

Edward Ellis III, Robert M. Kellman, and Emre Vural address questions for discussion and debate:

1. Are there specific indications for open versus closed treatment of subcondylar fractures? Are there any contraindications to open treatment, and do they supersede the indications for open treatment?

2. Does the presence of other fractures (mandible and/or midface) affect your choice of open versus closed treatment? (Is the selection of closed vs open treatment the same for unilateral vs bilateral fractures?)

3. If one chooses to perform closed treatment, how long a period of maxillomandibular fixation is required?

4. What are the most important factors for success when closed treatment is used?

5. What is the best surgical approach to open reduction and internal fixation of subcondylar fractures?

6. *Analysis:* Over the past 5 years, how has your technique or approach evolved and what is the most important thing you have learned/observed in working with subcondylar fractures?

Are there specific indications for open versus closed treatment of subcondylar fractures? Are there any contraindications to open treatment, and do they supersede the indications for open treatment?

ELLIS

I applaud this debate because I believe it is time we stopped arguing about whether condylar fractures should be treated open or closed, and instead ask which condylar fractures might have better outcomes when treated open.

I find it pejorative to come up with specific "indications" for open or closed treatment. I prefer to use the term "considerations," for which there are many. I can think of only 1 situation in which I believe open treatment should almost always be

---

[a] Department of Oral and Maxillofacial Surgery, The University of Texas Health Science Center at San Antonio, San Antonio, TX, USA
[b] Department of Otolaryngology-Head and Neck Surgery, University of Arkansas for Medical Sciences, 4301 West Markham, Slot 543, Little Rock, AR 72205, USA
[c] Department of Otolaryngology and Communication Sciences, State University of New York – Upstate Medical University, 750 East Adams Street, Syracuse, NY 13210, USA
* Corresponding authors.
E-mail addresses: ellise3@uthscsa.edu; kellmanr@upstate.edu; vuralemrea@uams.edu

Facial Plast Surg Clin N Am 20 (2012) 365–382
doi:10.1016/j.fsc.2012.05.002
1064-7406/12/$ – see front matter © 2012 Published by Elsevier Inc.

used, and it is addressed later (condylar fractures associated with comminuted maxillary fracture[s]). However, there are other considerations that may push one toward one treatment or the other and I address these now.

However, to fully understand condylar fractures, one has to understand the adaptations in the masticatory system that occur when these injuries are treated closed or open. I refer readers to an article on this topic by Ellis and Throckmorton.[2]

First, I believe that any unilateral condylar fracture can be treated closed, with the following prerequisites:

1. The patient must have a good complement of teeth, especially posterior teeth. Without them, there is a significant loss of posterior vertical dimension and an increase in the mandibular and occlusal plane angles. The loss of posterior vertical dimension makes future prosthetic reconstruction difficult.
2. The patient must be cooperative. They must wear their elastics, do their functional exercises, and return often for follow-up.
3. The surgeon must be willing to see the patient often to assess treatment and alter functional therapy as necessary.

It does not matter to me whether the unilateral condylar fracture is intracapsular, condylar neck, or subcondylar. Nor does the degree of displacement matter to me. (It does not matter to me if there is a condyle. Unilateral condylectomy patients can readily be treated nonsurgically with excellent outcomes.) They can all be managed effectively if the criteria listed earlier are met. However, one must understand completely that, when one chooses closed treatment, especially those with large displacements, the neoarticulation does not translate as much as the nonfractured side. The consequence of this situation in the skeletally mature patient is that they often deviate toward the side of fracture when the mouth is opened (see **Fig. 1**A in the techniques section) and they have limited lateral excursion away from the side of fracture (**Fig. 1**).[3–5] When they protrude their mandible, they also deviate toward the side of fracture. This deviation is not a failure of treatment; it is a consequence of the alteration in biomechanics secondary to the displaced condyle and the altered lateral pterygoid function. It is of no clinical consequence to the patient. That is not to say that patients treated open for unilateral condylar fractures do not do well. They usually do well, assuming that no injuries occur from the surgery to reduce and stabilize the condyle. However, one has to consider the risk/benefit ratio when deciding on treatment. If one can obtain a good

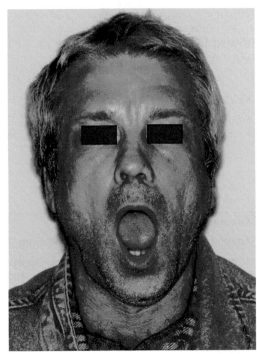

Fig. 1. A patient treated closed for a left condylar process fracture. Note the deviation toward the side of fracture.

occlusion, good facial symmetry, and pain-free function by treating someone closed, why should they risk the potential intraoperative and postoperative complications that are associated with open treatment?[1]

Unlike the unilateral condylar fracture, I do not believe that I can satisfactorily treat all bilateral condylar fractures closed. Some have good outcomes; some do not. The problem is that I cannot predict which ones will do well with closed treatment and which will not. The bilateral condylar fracture, especially those that are displaced, creates a biomechanical alteration that is a challenge to the masticatory system. Bilateral loss of vertical and horizontal support from disruption of the craniomandibular articulation means that the mandible is essentially a free-floating bone, positioned only by the muscles and ligaments attached to it, and the dentition.[1,6,7] Some patients have the neuromuscular ability to adapt to the alteration in biomechanics and others do not. A successful outcome requires the muscle coordination to be such that the patient can carry the mandible in the proper position while a new craniomandibular articulation is established. The reestablishment of a new articulation always occurs. The only question is whether the mandible will be in a favorable position at the conclusion of the process by which the neoarticulation is established. Because I cannot predict who will and will not readily adapt, I tend to treat bilateral condylar fractures, especially those that are displaced, by open reduction and internal fixation (ORIF) of at least one of the fractured condylar processes. However, the literature shows that perhaps only 10% of patients with bilateral condylar fractures develop malocclusions that are beyond the capability of orthodontic or prosthetic reconstruction, requiring orthognathic surgery.[8] It is always hard to recommend that 100% of patients should undergo open treatment of their condylar fractures when 90% of them do not need it. The clinicians need to keep this in mind. Again, it is the risk/benefit ratio of open versus closed treatment that must be considered.

When a patient has the combination of a very mobile, very comminuted maxillary fracture and condylar fracture(s), I usually perform ORIF of the condylar process fracture(s). I do this because with a panfacial fracture, I choose to reconstruct the mandible first. This procedure requires that all fractures of the mandible undergo open reduction and stable internal fixation. I essentially turn a panfacial fracture into an isolated midfacial fracture. When one has an isolated midface fracture, the nonfractured mandible serves as a platform on which the maxillary arch can be positioned through maxillomandibular fixation (MMF). Because the mandible still maintains its position with respect to the cranium through the craniomandibular articulation, using the mandible provides the proper mediolateral and anteroposterior position of the maxilla. The only dimension one needs to obtain at surgery is the vertical dimension, rotating the maxillomandibular complex around the temporomandibular joint (TMJ). When the mandibular condyle is also fractured and the mandible is used to position the maxilla, one must reestablish the continuity of the mandible. Otherwise, the midface is positioned off-midline because of the tendency of the mandible to deviate to the side of the condylar fracture. That is not to say that one must always treat a panfacial fracture in this manner. The other way is to stabilize the midfacial bones, including the maxilla, using bony interfaces as guides. Once stabilized, the condylar fracture could even be treated closed. However, in my experience, it is difficult to properly position the maxilla in all 3 planes of space when the bony articulations, especially those along the anterior maxilla, are comminuted.

Another injury for which one might consider the open treatment of condylar fracture(s) is the edentulous patient. As noted earlier, if the patient has no teeth, especially posterior teeth, it is difficult to prevent the posterior mandible from moving superiorly during the formation of the neoarticulation. Even with insertion of the patient's dentures, there is no evidence that they can prevent the tendency for loss of posterior vertical dimension. The consequence of that loss is difficulty in future prosthetic reconstruction. Treating condylar fracture(s) closed in such patients not only requires that they wear their dentures but that the dentures be secured to the jaws. Otherwise, there is no way to control the tendency for deviation of the mandible toward the side of a unilateral condylar fracture or the anterior open bite tendency in bilateral fractures. Performing open treatment in these patients allows them to go back to wearing dentures immediately.

A discussion on this topic is not complete without discussing the skeletal maturation of the patient. This is another major consideration for me. Every study in the literature that has studied this topic suggests that skeletally immature patients have a better ability to adapt to a condylar fracture than skeletally mature patients when treated closed (**Fig. 2**).[9–14] Therefore, there is less need to perform open treatment of condylar process fractures in young patients. That is not to say that open treatment is not also effective. However, it comes back to the risk/benefit ratio. The bone in the young does not always allow secure purchase for the bone screws. The last thing one would like is loose hardware in the wound. Therefore, before performing ORIF, one has to be able to convince oneself that open treatment provides better outcomes than closed treatment.

Several considerations must be entertained before open treatment is planned. First is the ability of the surgeon to obtain an anatomic

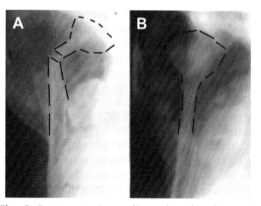

Fig. 2. Posteroanterior radiographs of a fractured mandibular condylar process in a 6-year-old child before (*A*) and 6 months after closed treatment (*B*). Note that it is almost impossible to determine that fracture had occurred.

reduction and stable internal fixation. If one cannot assure oneself that one is likely to be successful in this procedure, then closed treatment might be a better option. For instance, intracapsular or diacapitular fractures of the condyle are difficult to treat open. Those surgeons who are skilled in TMJ surgery may be able to predictably perform open reduction and internal derangement of such fractures, but many surgeons find this a challenging exercise. Therefore, for most surgeons who treat maxillofacial injuries, a relative contraindication is the intracapsular or diacapitular fracture.

Another consideration hinges on the surgical approach that one might use to perform ORIF. For those surgeons who use a transfacial approach, the ability to turn the head is critical to exposing the fracture. For patients with unstable cervical spine fractures or those in halo frames, the head cannot be turned. For surgeons who

use a transfacial approach, cervical spine fractures may therefore become a contraindication to open treatment. For those surgeons who use an approach that does not require the head to be turned (ie, the transoral approach), a cervical spine fracture is not a contraindication.

Another consideration for me is the patient with a condylar fracture who can still maintain a good occlusion, even when a posteriorly directed force is applied to the chin.[15] If, after application of arch bars and ORIF of other fractures of the mandible, the occlusion is stable and reproducible to manual manipulation with posteriorly directed force applied to the chin, I see no reason to perform ORIF of the condylar process fracture. Although fractured, the fragments provide good support to the anterior mandible.[15] These are the easiest cases to treat closed. For me, this is a relative contraindication to open treatment.

KELLMAN

The question assumes that the diagnosis of a subcondylar fracture (or of bilateral subcondylar fractures) has been made. However, if that diagnosis is made, one must still return to the issue of diagnosis. One of the first controversies that we face as clinicians is how to evaluate these injuries. Whereas some surgeons are satisfied with a panoramic tomographic radiograph (orthopantomogram), others suggest the benefit of plain films of the mandible, because the Towne view provides an excellent view of the vertical rami of the mandible, allowing assessment of angulation of the condylar segment, as well as assessment of the vertical height of the ramus-condyle unit. Schubert and colleagues have found that the combination of computed tomography (CT) scans and orthopantomograms provides the most complete diagnostic evaluation of mandibular fractures, and Lee and colleagues advocate obtaining both axial and coronal CT views of the ramus/condyle unit when subcondylar fractures are suspected.[1,2] These views show alterations in vertical height and angulation as well as rotation of the condylar segment. CT also provides for better assessment of comminution, although it often underestimates the extent of comminution.

Although the various radiographs provide for excellent analysis of the fracture, the most important assessment is clinical. If the patient is able to open and close normally or near-normally and achieve their normal occlusal relationship easily, then limited intervention is generally warranted. A soft diet along with early physiotherapy usually provides a satisfactory result. However, if there is

a shift in the chin point to one side or the other or if there is visible foreshortening of one side of the mandible (and therefore an alteration in facial appearance), or widening of the face because of malposition of the bone, then additional options should be discussed with the patient. Similarly, if the patient has difficulty bringing the teeth into a premorbid occlusal relationship, additional intervention is warranted.

Experience has shown that most subcondylar fractures of the mandible can be successfully managed using nonopen techniques. This statement does not mean that so-called closed techniques reduce subcondylar fractures. They do not. However, they do manage the occlusion, and most patients achieve what have long been considered satisfactory results using this approach. For me, closed management (I am not saying closed reduction) entails the application of arch bars to the upper and lower dentition followed by the use of limited elastic traction (commonly referred to as training elastics) to gently pull the dentition into a premorbid relationship and permit function, so that the patient can open and close the mouth. This strategy also allows for early physiotherapy. The elastics are left in place until the patient can maintain their premorbid occlusal relationship without them. This procedure requires close follow-up, particularly because the option of reconsidering open reduction for those patients for whom this approach is not working well should be considered earlier rather than later (preferably within 1 to 2 weeks). Probably the single biggest controversy in the management of these fractures is the question of when open reduction should be used, because some surgeons perform open reduction freely on most if not all fractures, whereas others use open reduction rarely if ever, and most fall somewhere between.

Open reduction should be performed when a reasonable occlusal relationship cannot be achieved, even under general anesthesia with muscle relaxation. It should also be considered for those patients who are bothered by the alteration (or, in discussion with the patient, the potential alteration) in their cosmetic appearance that results from the change in the mandibular shape. The presence of edema can make this alteration difficult to determine early on, and sometimes the likelihood or potential of these changes developing is part of the discussion with the patient, because the final appearance with and without surgery may be difficult to predict precisely in a timely fashion that allows for timely repair. The surgical repair of subcondylar fractures becomes more difficult as time passes, so it is often necessary to make a surgical decision before the swelling has gone down sufficiently for the patient to decide based on the appearance.

Open reduction can be performed transcutaneously with direct exposure of the fractured fragments, or it can be performed via a transoral approach, typically with the aid of an angled endoscope for better visualization of the fragments when using the transoral approach. The choice of surgical approach is yet another controversy.[3] Once the bone fragments are reduced, 1 or 2 titanium miniplates are generally applied across the fracture, although the size, strength, and number of plates required to obtain a good result are not clear and may even vary from patient to patient. When open reduction is used, I still prefer to apply arch bars and use the same postoperative approach that I use with closed management (ie, loose training elastics and physiotherapy).

As noted earlier, the foremost reason to perform open reduction of a subcondylar fracture of the mandible is the inability to reduce the occlusion, particularly if this inability persists under general anesthesia with muscle relaxation. If the patient cannot come into occlusion themselves, the surgeon may still be able to compensate for this under anesthesia, and if preferred by either the patient or the surgeon, closed management with training elastics and physiotherapy may still be attempted. However, when the occlusion cannot be reduced under anesthesia, a poor outcome is almost assured, and therefore open reduction is warranted to try to achieve a better functional result. Two recent prospective studies have suggested better outcomes when open surgical reduction and repair are used,[4,5] although there are conflicting data as well.[6] The study by Eckelt and colleagues[4] is particularly worthy of careful review, because the randomization was impressive, so that severity of injury was not used to determine the treatment, unlike the situation with almost all of the retrospective studies, which showed little difference regardless of treatment category. (In most of these reviews, the results of the open and closed treatments were similar despite the fact that the more severe fractures with more severe displacement/dysfunction were generally in the open groups.)

Cosmetic deformity is also an important consideration. When there is significant foreshortening on radiograph (>1 cm) (**Fig. 3**), the change in the patient's appearance may be apparent, although the amount of overlap that correlates with a noticeable cosmetic deformity has to my knowledge never been studied. However, it may be necessary to discuss the risk of cosmetic deformity with the patient, even when it is not yet apparent because of swelling. Because open reduction is not without its own attendant risks, the surgeon needs to be careful to inform rather than lead the patient.

The presence of midfacial fractures, particularly when severe enough to make determination of facial height challenging, should be considered an indication for open reduction. In this situation, the reestablishment of the vertical height of the ramus of the mandible serves as a guide to the midfacial position.[7] This situation leads directly to the next question.

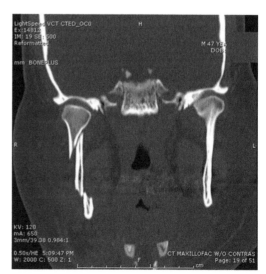

Fig. 3. A coronal CT scan showing a typical subcondylar fracture with lateral displacement of the proximal fragment and significant loss of vertical ramus height caused by overlap of the fragments.

When considering contraindications to open repair, any other medical condition that would contraindicate proceeding with anything other than life-or-death surgery should similarly be considered a contraindication. However, in terms of maxillofacial contraindications, I would expected failure, such as might be predicted with very high or severely comminuted fractures would be in this category. These are relative contraindications, though, and if there is a particular clinical indication for open reduction, it should probably supersede a contraindication in this category. However, just as the evolution of treatment from closed to open repair of subcondylar fractures is progressing, the same might be said for fractures of the condylar head. Most surgeons, particularly in the United States, see few if any indications for repairing condylar head fractures, but there is a small but increasing group of European surgeons who believe that open reduction of condylar head fractures yields better outcomes.[8,9] The absence of dentition makes closed management difficult, so if there is displacement or foreshortening that necessitates treatment, an open approach should be entertained. Although most surgeons rarely open subcondylar fractures in children younger than 14 years, age younger than this is not considered an absolute contraindication.

VURAL

Although there is almost universal consensus on the management of pediatric subcondylar fractures, which are almost exclusively treated with a closed approach, treatment of subcondylar mandibular fractures in the adult population probably forms one of the most controversial topics of discussion in maxillofacial trauma. Therefore, it is difficult to establish absolute indications or contraindications for open versus closed management of these fractures. Use of an endoscopic approach in the treatment of subcondylar fractures is an exciting recent advance.[1,2] However, the question of whether these fractures need to be managed closed or open still exists. I believe that both approaches have a role in the management of subcondylar fractures and each of these approaches may serve better than the other in certain conditions.

The goal in the treatment of subcondylar fractures should be providing the patient with a satisfactory occlusion with the least possible discomfort and limitation of movement in the mandible. However, the jury is still out on deciding which approach is the best to accomplish this goal, because there are no high-quality published data comparing of the outcomes of closed, open, or endoscopic management of subcondylar fractures. A recent Cochrane review performed by Sharif and colleagues[3] indicates that the decision of which is the best approach in subcondylar fractures may not be made based on current evidence. Another recent study performed by Nussbaum and colleagues,[4] which involved a meta-analysis of published data on condylar fractures in adults, revealed that most of the parameters showed no difference between open and closed approaches, although some parameters favored one approach over another. As stated in these 2 articles,[3,4] there are numerous shortcomings in the presentation of the published data on subcondylar fractures; such as lack of uniformity in patient populations, bias in the selection of approach, and subjective evaluation of certain parameters. When we present data on occlusion for open and closed approaches, do we really know how the occlusion was for any given patient before the event causing the fracture? Do we pick and choose what we plate and what we do not plate? And, do we really know if one particular patient treated with one approach would do the same, better, or worse if the other approach was used?

An exhaustive literature review in this topic reveals both significant and nonsignificant differences between open and closed approaches, for almost all parameters, such as occlusion, excursion, pain, interincisal opening, protrusion, or deviation.[5–12] Considering all these, it is impossible to establish absolute indications for each treatment approach. Fracture of the subcondylar region is an unfortunate event, and both good and bad outcomes are possibilities regardless of the approach chosen. Multiple other factors are involved in obtaining the final outcome (satisfactory or unsatisfactory) in any given patient, in addition to the selected management approach. The status of the patient's dentition, compliance, bone stock quality, age, comorbid conditions, occlusal relationship before the event causing fracture, and presence of additional maxillofacial fractures, infection, or other accompanying life-threatening issues such as intracranial injuries are just a few. Therefore, it is more appropriate to talk about personal preferences rather than indications/contraindications of open versus closed treatment.

Nonetheless, performing open or endoscopic reduction/fixation in a subcondylar fracture may be contraindicated if the patient is not a candidate for general anesthesia, does not wish to undergo open or endoscopic surgery, or has other life-threatening issues to be resolved. The benefits of attempting rigid fixation of high fractures such as intracapsular fractures or condylar head fractures are questionable and may not outweigh the risks. Therefore, rigid fixation may be considered contraindicated in these fractures.

Does the presence of other fractures (mandible or midface) affect your choice of open versus closed treatment? (Is the selection of closed vs open treatment the same for unilateral vs bilateral fractures?)

ELLIS

I addressed these issues fully in my first response. To summarize, I believe that any unilateral condylar fracture can be treated closed, with several prerequisites. Unlike the unilateral condylar fracture, I do not believe that I can satisfactorily treat all bilateral condylar fractures closed. Some have good outcomes; some do not. The problem is that I cannot predict which ones will do well with closed treatment and which will not. It is always difficult to recommend that 100% of patients should undergo open treatment of their condylar fractures when 90% of them do not need it. Clinicians need to keep this in mind. Again, the risk/benefit ratio of open versus closed treatment must be considered.

KELLMAN

As noted earlier, the presence of severe midfacial fractures usually requires direct (open) repair of displaced subcondylar fractures. When the midface is comminuted, the mandible serves as a template for positioning of the alveolus, thereby determining the relationship of the maxillary dental arches to the remainder of the face and skull. Foreshortening of the mandibular height as a result of loss of continuity of the ramus-condyle unit positions the maxillary dental arches superiorly, with resultant foreshortening of the midface (in essence, an accidental maxillary intrusion).

One should also consider the presence of other mandible fractures. In particular, the presence of symphyseal/parasymphyseal fractures of the mandible should be considered, because the combination of these fractures is a setup for widening of the mandible with lingual splaying of the symphyseal fracture(s). It is difficult to adequately reduce the symphyseal region first, and therefore, I prefer to open and repair the subcondylar fracture(s) first, before applying the final fixation to the symphysis (**Fig. 4**). For this type of combination, bilateral subcondylar fractures are more difficult than unilateral, although widening can result with a unilateral fracture as well.

On the other hand, the presence of bilateral subcondylar fractures in isolation does not mandate an open repair, and this situation can often be managed with the same approach as a unilateral fracture.

VURAL

Presence of other fractures in the mandible or in the midface does not affect my choice of treatment of the subcondylar fracture(s). I do not feel obliged to plate one fracture (if it is suitable to be managed by conservative approach), just because I plate the other. The condition of the other fractures, rather than their presence, is important, because some midface fractures or selected fractures of other sites of the mandible could easily be managed by a conservative approach in the form of a soft diet. For example, if a nondisplaced tripod fracture is managed by soft diet only, an accompanying nondisplaced subcondylar fracture with unaffected occlusion can also be managed by soft diet and should not be considered as a reason to operate. On the other hand, if the patient has multiple fractures, which need to be managed by ORIF, and if I believe that the subcondylar component could also benefit from an internal fixation; then I try to plate them all. Sometimes I apply arch bars with elastic bands for the subcondylar component in combination with applying plates and screws for the other fractures in the face. Therefore, a patient may have ORIF or closed management in all facial fracture components, as well as ORIF in some and closed management for others.

Similarly, having a unilateral or bilateral subcondylar fracture should not affect the decision-making process in the management of

A **B** **C**

D **E**

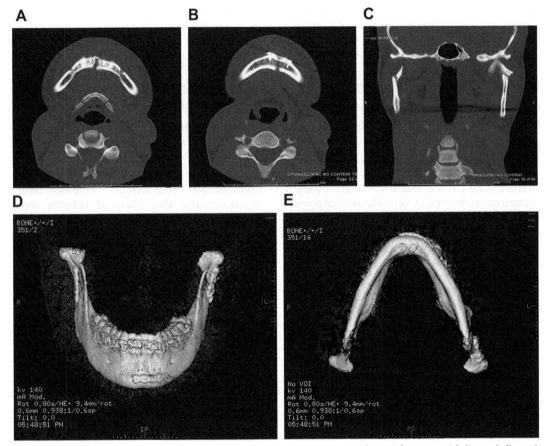

Fig. 4. (A) Axial CT scan of the anterior mandibular body showing a symphyseal fracture with lingual diastasis. What is not apparent is that this patient has had an attempt at repair (see B). (B) Same CT scan as in (A), but the CT cut shows that a plate has been placed. However, bilateral subcondylar fractures have not been addressed (see C). (C) Coronal CT scan showing bilateral subcondylar fractures with the distal ramus segments directed laterally out of the glenoid fossae. (D) Three-dimensional (3D) CT scan reconstruction after secondary repair, including plating of both subcondylar fractures, allowing better control of the symphyseal fracture. (E) Same 3D CT scan rotated to show the mandible from the inferior view, showing closure of the lingual cortex of the symphyseal fracture.

subcondylar fractures. Whereas nondisplaced bilateral subcondylar fractures can be managed by soft diet only if the occlusion is not affected, a displaced unilateral fracture with malocclusion is best treated with an elastic MMF or open approach. Therefore, occlusal status plays a more important role in decision making, rather than the fracture being unilateral versus bilateral.

If one chooses to perform closed treatment, how long a period of maxillomandibular fixation is required?

ELLIS

I do not use postoperative MMF for patients who are treated closed for fractures of the mandibular condylar process. Although doing so is not contraindicated, there is no convincing evidence that it is helpful. There is good evidence that it is more useful to allow the patient to function immediately.[16–18] Patients allowed to do so increase their range of mandibular motion faster, and their speech, diet, and oral hygiene are facilitated.

Instead, I use aggressive physiotherapy and control of the occlusion by 1 or 2 interarch elastics in a class II direction on the side of fracture. The patient is weaned off the elastics over the 4 to 6 weeks after arch bars have been applied.[1]

KELLMAN

I generally no longer use rigid MMF in the management of subcondylar fractures. The exception is the rare situation in which I have performed an open reduction, but for some technical reason, I have been unable to apply any rigid fixation hardware. In this situation, I place the patient in rigid MMF for 10 days to discourage displacement of the now reduced but not fixated fracture fragments. However, despite the logic of this approach, there is no good evidence that it is successful. Raveh and colleagues[10,11] reported success with this technique, but it seems that the proximal fragment likely displaces secondary to muscle pull, even with the jaws immobilized in MMF.

I like the idea of early functioning of the mandible to improve the likelihood of better functional outcomes, although the belief that poor function is caused by prolonged MMF has never been proved either. It is likely that the joint injury that occurs as a result of the initial trauma is the most meaningful predictor of later joint dysfunction. Nonetheless, because there is no evidence that early functioning interferes with the outcome, this approach at least makes intuitive sense. Early physiotherapy should be able to increase range of motion of the mandible in all directions, whereas the elastics provide the guidance to train the muscles to bring the dentition into the best occlusal relationship, despite the malposition of unreduced bone fragments.

VURAL

I believe that there is a consensus on keeping the MMF as short as possible.[13] Long-term rigid MMF can cause ankylosis in the TMJ, which can cause limitation in the range of motion. If I could bring the patient into satisfactory occlusion with elastic bands, I would choose not to use rigid MMF using wires. In this case, I would closely follow the patient and try to eliminate elastic bands over the next 3 to 4 weeks. If the patient fell into a correct occlusal relationship without elastic bands and maintains this relationship, I would remove the arch bars. If I could bring the patient into satisfactory occlusion only by using rigid MMF using wires, I would keep these wires for only 1 or 2 weeks and switch to training elastics, as I mentioned in my second response.

What are the most important factors for success when closed treatment is used?

ELLIS

My full response to this is within the first question; however, it bears repeating, I believe that any unilateral condylar fracture can be treated closed with prerequisites:

1. The patient must have a good complement of teeth, especially posterior teeth. Without them, there is a significant loss of posterior vertical dimension and an increase in the mandibular and occlusal plane angles. The loss of posterior vertical dimension makes future prosthetic reconstruction difficult.

2. The patient must be cooperative. They must wear their elastics, do their functional exercises, and return often for follow-up.
3. The surgeon must be willing to see the patient often to assess treatment and alter functional therapy as necessary.

For a successful outcome for bilateral condylar fractures treated closed, the risk/benefit ratio of open versus closed treatment must be considered.

Patient muscle coordination

Patient muscle coordination requires that the muscle coordination is such that patients can carry the mandible in the proper position while a new craniomandibular articulation is established.

Once midfacial bones and maxilla are stabilized in patients with combination of a very mobile, very comminuted maxillary fracture and condylar fracture(s), the condylar fracture could even be treated closed. However, in my experience, it is difficult to properly position the maxilla in all 3 planes of space when the bony articulations, especially those along the anterior maxilla, are comminuted.

Dentition

Without teeth, especially posterior teeth, it is difficult to prevent the posterior mandible from moving superiorly during the formation of the neoarticulation.

Performing open treatment in edentulous patients allows them to go back to wearing dentures immediately.

Skeletal maturity

There is less need to perform open treatment of condylar process fractures in young patients. That

is not to say that open treatment is not also effective. However, it comes back to the risk/benefit ratio.

KELLMAN

First, it is important to define success when closed management is chosen as the treatment of subcondylar fractures. If there is foreshortening of the mandible on the side of a subcondylar fracture, the use of closed management is not likely to resolve this. However, that statement to some extent begs an important question: how often is foreshortening significant, and the obvious corollary question is that when it is significant, to whom is it significant: the patient or the astute cosmetically oriented surgeon (or both)? Like so many issues in medicine, many examples of facial foreshortening are not noticed by the patient until the surgeon points it out. This is a difficult situation, because it is unclear whether it is more ethical to point it out to the patient in the interest of full disclosure and risk creating dissatisfaction with the self-image where none existed, or whether ethics suggest that we should not create concern when the patient does not independently raise the issue. I do not know how to resolve this issue, but my personal

approach is to mention the risk of facial foreshortening (in general terms as a risk of this type of fracture) during my initial discussion with the patient and then be guided by the level of concern that the patient then expresses. If the patient finds this to be a concern, and there is significant overlap (foreshortening) on the radiograph, then I think the option of reestablishing ramus height via open reduction must be candidly discussed with the patient.

Another key factor in obtaining a good result is patient compliance. It is difficult to expect a good functional outcome when the patient is not willing to be an active partner in their care. A patient who removes the elastics (possibly even the arch bars) and fails to comply with exercises or physiotherapy sessions is less likely to obtain the best possible outcome. There is no way to ensure patient compliance with our treatment regimens, and we have to do our best to educate patients as to how important their participation is in the final result.

VURAL

In my opinion, one of the most important factors in successful management of subcondylar fractures is the presence or absence of malocclusion. I believe that patients with unilateral or bilateral subcondylar fracture(s) with normal occlusal relationship may do better than the ones who present with malocclusion; and the ones with malocclusion that can be easily corrected with elastics do better than the ones with malocclusion that cannot be corrected with elastics and necessitates rigid MMF. Some patients may have malocclusion as a result of fractures of other mandibular sites or midface. If normal occlusion is obtained by performing ORIF on those other fracture sites in the presence of 1 or 2 subcondylar fractures, these patients may still do well in the long term,

if the subcondylar component is appropriately managed.

Another important factor is the patient's compliance. A nondisplaced or minimally displaced subcondylar fracture can be easily and optimally managed by keeping the patient on a soft diet only, if the patient is compliant with the regimen. Conversely, a patient who was kept on excellent occlusion on elastic MMF may lose this occlusal relationship easily and quickly, for example, if broken elastics are not replaced in a timely fashion.

One other important factor is the level of the fracture, because I believe that the outcome becomes worse as the level of fracture gets higher (ie, low subcondylar vs intracapsular fractures).

What is the best surgical approach to open reduction internal fixation of subcondylar fractures?

ELLIS

I prefer the retromandibular approach.[19] It provides direct access to the entire posterior ramus and condylar neck, and can be performed rapidly. The problem with the preauricular approach is that it gives good exposure of the TMJ but poor exposure of the subcondylar region. Placing a bone plate through this approach is difficult because insertion of the screws below the fracture requires some inferior retraction of the facial nerve. The problem with the submandibular approach is that it is positioned a long way away from the fractured condylar process. One therefore must work down a long tunnel. Placing screws may therefore require a transcutaneous trochar, especially for the screws above the fracture. I occasionally use a transoral approach with endoscopic assistance, but I am not expert in this approach so I cannot predictably attain a good reduction and stable internal fixation. For surgeons skilled in the transoral approach, it is ideal because the scar is hidden and the anatomic hazards (ie, nerves and vessels) are largely avoided.

KELLMAN

There are several approaches to the ramus/subcondylar region of the mandible, and each surgeon should use the approach with which they are most comfortable. Most surgeons articulate the reasons that they prefer their particular approach.

My favorite surgical approach is the endoscope-assisted transoral approach, with the use of a transbuccal stab incision for placement of screws into the plate or plates that are used to fixate the fracture. Although it takes longer to perform this approach when one is less experienced, there is good evidence that the duration of these procedures decreases as experience is gained.[12] The advantages include minimizing the external scar (the procedure can be performed completely transorally using a right-angled drill and screwdriver, in which case there is not even the tiny scar associated with the transbuccal stab incision), and the risk of facial nerve injury seems to be less.[3,12] The incision for this approach is made along the anterior ramus of the mandible by feeling the bone and cutting directly down to it with an electrocautery wand. For greater visualization of the vertical ramus when needed, the incision can be extended inferiorly along the oblique line, as might be done for intraoral management of mandibular angle fractures. The elevation is performed in the subperiosteal plane, between the masseter muscle and the bone. As the elevation is performed, care must be taken not to elevate superiorly into the joint space, medial to the proximal fragment, which is more commonly laterally displaced. Once the elevation is completed, fracture reduction is accomplished by applying inferior traction on the posterior mandible, thereby allowing reduction of the proximal fragment into the space superior to the ramus. After reduction is accomplished, fixation may be applied. When I am unable to successfully perform the ORIF via this approach I either convert to a transcutaneous approach or I see if open reduction without fixation allows reduction of the occlusion and use of closed management. When I do convert to a transcutaneous open procedure, I prefer the submandibular approach, which allows for visualization of the mandibular ramus of the facial nerve to protect it, and avoidance of the parotid gland, which is sectioned when using the retromandibular approach. However, for high subcondylar fractures, the submandibular approach does require some retraction, which can be a source of stretch injury to the main trunk of the facial nerve.

The transoral approach may be helpful in reducing medially displaced proximal fragments, because it is possible to perform an elevation on the medial (lingual) side of the ramus of the mandible. The medially displaced proximal fragment can then be directly visualized or the endoscope may be used. Once it is exposed, an instrument or a finger may be used to carry out the lateral repositioning and reduction of the fragment. Care should be taken when dissecting in this area.

VURAL

I believe that the endoscopic approach is probably the best open approach for subcondylar fractures. I believe that most subcondylar fractures can be plated with the endoscopic approach, if they are suitable for plating. If the fracture is low enough to accommodate a 2-mm plate with at least 2 screw holes on each side of the fracture and the fracture is fresh enough to allow manipulation of the proximal segment (ie, a maximum of 7–10 days old), the preauricular approach is not indicated most of the time, and equally satisfactory reduction and

fixation can be performed with endoscopic approach.

Analysis: Over the past 5 years, how has your technique or approach evolved and what is the most important thing you have learned/observed in working with subcondylar fractures?

ELLIS

I have not changed my technique for closed or open treatment of condylar process fractures in more than 20 years. I believe that I have a good feel for which cases can be treated closed, which might do better treated open, and how to provide that treatment.

KELLMAN

Over the last decade, my approach has changed significantly, both in regard to closed management as well as my approach to ORIF. A decade ago, I was still leaning toward more closed treatments and fewer open reductions. Furthermore, the closed treatments were more generally referred to as closed reductions, although most surgeons were aware that it was the occlusion rather than the fracture that was being reduced. I now make a point of clarifying that difference, both to patients as well as to other members of the health care delivery team. Having become involved early in the use of the endoscopic-assisted open reduction approaches, I overcame my initial reluctance to accept the possibility of frequent open reduction for a fracture that I had almost always treated with closed management, with what at the time had seemed like satisfactory results. Although for me, it may have been the use of the endoscope that led to this shift, it was also a timely shift, because more and more surgeons seem to be recognizing that reducing the fractures, rather than accepting forced adaptation of the occlusion despite nonreduced fractures, may provide better outcomes in many cases. Perhaps the reluctance to open these fractures in previous years[13] was partly because of unacceptably high complications, particularly the dreaded seventh nerve palsy, which probably led to surgeons' discomfort with open reduction. Other factors probably played a role as well. However, with better surgical techniques, the incidence of facial nerve injury seems to be less of a concern, and more surgeons are advocating ORIF.

The other major evolution has been in how I manage my closed management patients. When I trained, we were using rigid MMF with wire for 6 weeks, probably because of the mistaken belief at the time that we were reducing the fractures by this effort, and therefore we needed to put the jaw at rest so that it could heal. Over time, I found myself using shorter and shorter periods of rigid MMF, until the last 5 to 10 years, when I progressed to the approach indicated earlier, using training elastics and physiotherapy, with few remaining indications for rigid MMF.

I would like to close by mentioning again what I believe is going to be the next frontier in this area. For years, even those who advocated ORIF of subcondylar fractures[7] advocated avoiding direct repair of the condylar head. Most recently, a small but increasing group of surgeons are performing ORIF on many condylar head fractures.[8,9] Although this is probably the newest area of controversy in the management of mandible fractures, it is not unlikely that the trend toward opening many of these fractures will increase in the future.

VURAL

My approach was almost exclusively closed at the beginning. Then, I did have a transition period, when I used endoscopic ORIF as much as possible. I finally settled on a blend of endoscopic and closed management.

I do not think that plating is required in every subcondylar fracture, regardless of how suitable the fracture is for plating. A nondisplaced or minimally displaced subcondylar fracture with unaffected occlusion (ie, occlusion that did not change after trauma regardless of whether the occlusion is ideal or not) can easily be managed by close observation with the patient on a soft diet. If the fracture is causing malocclusion and seems to be suitable for an endoscopic ORIF, this may serve as an indication to operate, with the patient consenting to both open and closed management. If the proximal segment is large enough to accommodate at least 2 screws and the occlusion can be restored easily under general anesthesia by manual MMF, then an endoscopic ORIF should be attempted. In my opinion, providing correct occlusion easily by performing manual MMF under general anesthesia is a good predictor of maintenance of correct occlusion with elastic MMF (either with MMF screws or arch bars) during endoscopic ORIF.[14] If the occlusion can be restored with elastics, but the fracture is not suitable for plating or rigid fixation cannot be accomplished; then the patient is left on arch bars and training elastics. If the patient has malocclusion and the correct occlusion can be maintained only by applying rigid MMF, I typically avoid rigid fixation because rigid MMF may not allow manipulation of the distal fragment, which may be necessary for optimal reduction in the fracture line. An exception to this situation is the cases in which the proximal fragment can be reduced optimally, without the need for any manipulation of the distal mandible; I find this condition to be rare. In cases in which malocclusion can be corrected only with rigid MMF, I keep MMF wires for a week or 2 and replace these MMF wires with elastic bands as soon as possible.

If the patient has bilateral subcondylar fractures, I follow the same approach that has been explained earlier. It may be better to provide rigid fixation to at least 1 side, if it is possible, to prevent chronic anterior open bite as a result of premature contact of molar regions in bilateral fractures, if the patient has malocclusion. Some practitioners consider bilateral subcondylar fractures as an indication for open approach, with the fear that the patient will have shortening of the posterior facial length; however, I have not seen such a patient in my practice, probably because of masking of facial soft tissues of such skeletal deformities, unless the patient has significant anterior open bite.

If the patient is edentulous, but the occlusion is maintained when the dentures are in place, a nondisplaced or minimally displaced subcondylar fracture can be managed by a soft diet. If the denture-based occlusion is shifted because of significant displacement, and the fracture is suitable to be plated with the endoscopic approach, the best possible fracture reduction should be attempted by using endoscopic assistance. The patient can then be referred for new dentures or for adjustment of their old dentures. When the patient is edentulous and there is also senile atrophy in the mandible, the surgeon and the patient should be aware that the bone stock quality might not be good enough to maintain rigid fixation in the subcondylar region. Furthermore, stripping off the periosteum to obtain rigid fixation may cause disruption of the vascular supply to the bony fragments. Because the subcondylar region bears a significant amount of load because of the short distance of the fracture line to the fulcrum point (TMJ), loose hardware can be a complication in such patients.

Considering all of my past experiences, I can still say that most subcondylar fractures can be and should be managed with a closed approach.

Surgical techniques for subcondylar fracture

Edward Ellis' technique for closed treatment[1]

When the decision is made to treat the patient's condylar process fracture closed, the following steps are used:

1. Arch bars are applied.

2. Other (noncondylar) fractures are exposed.

3. Other (noncondylar) fractures are reduced and MMF is applied.

4. Stable internal fixation is applied to noncondylar fractures.

5. MMF is removed and the occlusion is examined. Typically, the mandible deviates toward the side of the condylar fracture (see **Fig. 1A, B**). This is of no consequence, and occlusal guidance commences the next day.

6. Placement of elastics as needed: the next day, the occlusion is assessed. Most commonly, there is a premature contact posteriorly on the side of the condylar process fracture. The mandible deviates to that side to varying degrees, with a resulting malocclusion. Occasionally, the patient is able to occlude normally without the use of guiding elastics. In this instance, they should be allowed to do so. If there is a malocclusion, elastics are applied to assist their neuromusculature to obtain the proper occlusion. For most unilateral fractures, this process is typically 1 elastic on the side of the condylar process fracture applied in a class II manner, to help draw the mandible anteriorly. Occasionally, a second one is necessary (see **Fig. 1C**). One should apply as much elastic guidance as is necessary to allow the patient to obtain their normal occlusal relationship when they occlude. However, the goal is to use as little as necessary to promote active use of the mandible. For bilateral fractures, elastics are usually required bilaterally in a class II vector, and often supplementation with vertical elastics in the anterior is necessary.

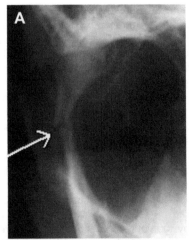

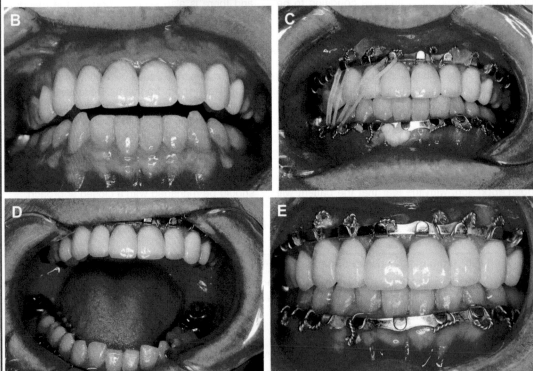

Fig. 1. Patient treated closed for right condylar neck fracture. (*A*) Posteroanterior radiograph showing fracture. (*B*) Preoperative occlusion with deviation to the side of the fracture (*right*). (*C*) Class II elastics placed on the side of the fracture (*right*), allowing establishment of the proper occlusal relationship. (*D*) 4 weeks after treatment, the patient can open widely. However, notice that the mandible deviates toward the side of fracture (*right*). (*E*) At 4 weeks, the patient's pretrauma occlusion is reestablished without the need for elastics. The arch bars can now be removed.

7. Postsurgical physiotherapy: patients are encouraged to use their jaws as much as possible beginning on the first postoperative day. They are instructed in physiotherapeutic exercises to increase range of mandibular motion, which they should perform at least 4 times a day. Exercises consist of maximum opening of the mouth, attempting to do so without deviation toward the side of fracture. This exercise can be facilitated by observing themselves in a mirror. The patient should also be shown how to use lateral excursive exercises to both the right and left sides. Protrusive excursions should be practiced, again attempting to do so without deviation of the mandible. During the exercises, eating, and oral hygiene procedures, the patient can remove the elastics. The elastics are then reapplied, and the

patient is shown how to determine that they are biting in the proper occlusal relationship in a mirror using as few elastics as possible. At bedtime, more elastics are used so that mandibular immobilization (MMF) is firmly established while sleeping. The elastics are removed in the morning for oral hygiene, breakfast, and exercises, and the patient then reapplies the minimum number of elastics as necessary to help them establish their proper occlusion when their teeth are occluded. The goal of physiotherapy should be an interincisal opening of greater than 40 mm, lateral excursions greater than 10 mm, and protrusive excursions greater than 5 mm. Patients with unilateral fractures may always have some degree of deviation toward the side of fracture on wide opening or protrusion (see **Fig. 1D**). Typically, patients are able to obtain the above treatment goals in 4 to 5 weeks.

8. Weaning the patient from use of elastics: after 2 or 3 weeks of this treatment, the patient should be able to obtain their pretraumatic occlusion without the constant use of elastics. The elastics are withdrawn more and more over the next 2 to 3 weeks so that they are used only while sleeping for another 2 to 3 weeks. Once the use of elastics is no longer necessary for the patient to obtain their pretraumatic occlusion, they can be discontinued (see **Fig. 1E**). However, the arch bars should be left in place for a few weeks beyond that time so that if the patient has some difficulty with occlusion later, elastics can be reapplied.

9. Removal of arch bars: most commonly, arch bars are left in place for 6 to 8 weeks for unilateral and 3 to 4 months for bilateral condylar process fractures. Once the patient can consistently assume their normal occlusion without the use of elastics, and they are no longer necessary for the patient to obtain their pretraumatic occlusion, the arch bars can be removed.

Edward Ellis' technique for open treatment[1]

When the decision is made to treat the patient's condylar process fracture with ORIF, the following steps are used:

1. Arch bars are applied.

2. Other (noncondylar) fractures are exposed.

3. Other (noncondylar) fractures are reduced and MMF is applied.

4. Stable internal fixation is applied to noncondylar fractures.

5. Placement of interarch elastics: before opening the condylar process fracture, the wire MMF is replaced with elastics. Enough elastics are placed between the upper and lower arch bars to provide the proper occlusal relationship. Elastics are used instead of wires during open treatment of the condylar process fractures because the mandibular ramus must frequently be distracted inferiorly to retrieve a medially displaced condylar process. The elastics allow this procedure, and on release of the distracting force, the proper occlusal relationship is again reestablished by the elastic force (**Fig. 2**).

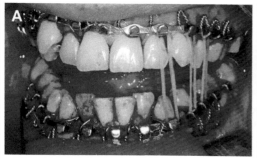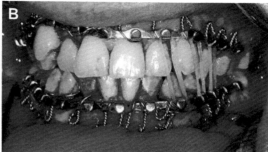

Fig. 2. Intraoperative photographs of a patient who will undergo ORIF of a left condylar process fracture. (*A*) Elastics are placed that have sufficient strength to allow reestablishment of the proper occlusion on release of the mandible (*B*) after forceful opening.

6. Open reduction of the condylar process fracture: the technique I describe uses a retromandibular, transparotid dissection to the posterior ramus. The incision for the retromandibular approach begins 0.5 cm below the lobe of the ear and continues inferiorly 2.5 to 3 cm (**Fig. 3A**). It is placed just behind the posterior border of the mandible and usually does not extend inferiorly below the level of the

mandibular angle. The skin is undermined to facilitate closure. Another incision is then made through the scant platysma muscle found in this location and the parotid capsule. At this point, blunt dissection begins in an anteromedial direction toward the posterior border of the mandible. The marginal mandibular and cervical branches of the facial nerve are frequently encountered during this dissection. A nerve stimulator can be used to identify branches of the facial nerve. When the buccal or marginal mandibular branches are located, they should be dissected free from surrounding tissues proximally for 1 cm and distally for 1.5 to 2 cm. Once the nerves are retracted, one can readily expose the pterygomasseteric sling at the posterior border of the mandible. One should also be cognizant of the retromandibular vein, which runs vertically in the same plane of dissection and is commonly exposed along its entire retromandibular course. This vein rarely requires ligation unless inadvertently transected. The periosteum along the posterior border of the mandible and partially around the mandibular angle is incised from as far superiorly as is reachable to as far inferiorly around the gonial angle as is possible. The masseter muscle is then stripped from the ramus. The fractured condylar fragment is then identified (see **Fig. 3**B) and reduced. This procedure may be more difficult for medially displaced fragments. A wire placed around a bone screw in the gonial angle may be useful to distract the mandibular ramus inferiorly during the dissection and retrieval of the fragment (see **Fig. 3**C).

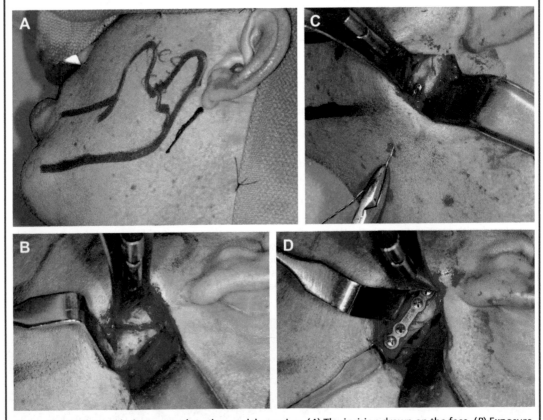

Fig. 3. The retromandibular approach to the condylar region. (*A*) The incision drawn on the face. (*B*) Exposure of the fracture. (*C*) A wire is inserted through the skin below the angle of the mandible and attached to a bone screw in the angle region to allow distraction of the ramus inferiorly to help retrieve a displaced condylar fragment. (*D*) Bone plate applied.

7. Reduction and stable internal fixation of condylar process fracture: the technique I routinely use is the application of a single strong bone plate using 2.0-mm self-threading screws (see **Fig. 3**D). One should use a bone plate of sufficient thickness because the standard miniplates using 2.0-mm screws readily fracture under function.

8. Occlusal verification: the occlusion is checked to ensure the mandible rotates properly into occlusion with the maxilla.

9. Closure: the incision is closed in layers, taking care to hermetically close the parotid capsule.

10. Occlusal guidance: the next day, assessment of the occlusion is performed. Most commonly, there is a slight posterior open bite on the side of the condylar process fracture. This open bite is usually secondary to edema in the TMJ and usually resolves within a week. If the posterior open bite is still present at the end of 1 week, light vertical elastics are applied to close the bite. Most commonly, the patient is able to occlude normally without the use of guiding elastics. In this instance, they should be allowed to do so. Elastics should be placed only if there is a malocclusion, and as few as necessary are used. The goal is to use as few as necessary to promote active use of the mandible.

11. Postsurgical physiotherapy: same as for closed treatment.

12. Removal of arch bars: once the patient can consistently assume their normal occlusion without the use of elastics, and they are no longer necessary for the patient to obtain their pretraumatic occlusion, the arch bars can be removed. Most commonly, arch bars are left in place for 4 to 6 weeks for condylar process fractures.

REFERENCES (ELLIS)

1. Ellis E. Condylar process fractures of the mandible. Facial Plast Surg 2000;16:193–205.
2. Ellis E, Throckmorton GS. Treatment of mandibular condylar process fractures: biological considerations. J Oral Maxillofac Surg 2005;63:115–34.
3. Amaratunga NA. A study of condylar fractures in Sri Lankan patients with special reference to the recent views on treatment, healing and sequelae. Br J Oral Maxillofac Surg 1987;25:391.
4. Palmieri C, Ellis E, Throckmorton GS. Mandibular motion after closed and open treatment of unilateral condylar process fractures. J Oral Maxillofac Surg 1999;57:764–75.
5. Throckmorton GS, Ellis E, Hayasaki H. Masticatory motion after surgical or non-surgical treatment for unilateral fractures of the mandibular condylar process. J Oral Maxillofac Surg 2004;62:127–38.
6. Choi BH. Comparison of computed tomography imaging before and after functional treatment of bilateral condylar fractures in adults. Int J Oral Maxillofac Surg 1996;25:30–3.
7. Talwar RW, Ellis E, Throckmorton GS. Adaptations of the masticatory system after bilateral fractures of the mandibular condylar process. J Oral Maxillofac Surg 1998;56:430–9.
8. Newman L. A clinical evaluation of the long-term outcome of patients treated for bilateral fracture of the mandibular condyles. Br J Oral Maxillofac Surg 1998;36:176–9.
9. Gilhuus-Möe O. Fractures of mandibular condyle in the growth period. Oslo (Norway): Universitetförlaget; 1969.
10. Gilhuus-Möe O. Fractures of the mandibular condyle: a clinical and radiographic examination of 62 patients injured in the growth period. In: Walker RV, editor. Oral surgery–transactions of the 3rd International Conference on Oral Surgery. Edinburgh (Scotland): E&S Livingstone; 1970. p. 121–9.
11. Lund K. Mandibular growth and remodeling processes after condylar fracture. Acta Odontol Scand Suppl 1974;32(64):75.
12. Lindahl L, Hollender L. Condylar fractures of the mandible. II. Radiographic study of remodeling processes in the temporomandibular joint. Int J Oral Surg 1977;6:153.
13. Bjuggren G. Fem fall av Käkortopediskt behandlade, enkelsidiga frakturer av collum mandibulae hos barn. Svenst Tandlaek T 1950;43:21 [in Swedish].
14. Kivimäki J, Ekholm A. Nachuntersuchungen von Brüchen des Kiefergelenkfortsatzes. Dtsch Zahn Mund Kierferheilkd Zentralbl 1959;31:139 [in German].
15. Ellis E. Method to determine when open treatment of condylar process fractures is not necessary. J Oral Maxillofac Surg 2009;67:1685–90.
16. Amaratunga NA. Mouth opening after release of MMF in fracture patients. J Oral Maxillofac Surg 1987;45:383.
17. Oikarinen KS, Raustia AM, Lahti J. Signs and symptoms of TMJ dysfunction in patients with mandibular condyle fractures. Cranio 1991;9:58.
18. Throckmorton GS, Ellis E. Recovery of mandibular motion after closed and open treatment of unilateral mandibular condylar process fractures. Int J Oral Maxillofac Surg 2000;29:421–7.
19. Ellis E, Dean J. Rigid fixation of mandibular condyle fractures. Oral Surg Oral Med Oral Pathol 1993;76:6–15.

REFERENCES (VURAL)

1. Kellman RM, Cienfuegos R. Endoscopic approaches to subcondylar fractures of the mandible. Facial Plast Surg 2009;25(1):23–8.
2. Vural E. Treatment of adult subcondylar mandibular fractures. Closed vs open vs endoscopic approach. Arch Otolaryngol Head Neck Surg 2004;130:1228–30.

3. Sharif MO, Fedorowicz Z, Drews P, et al. Intervention for the treatment of fractures of the mandibular condyle. Cochrane Database Syst Rev 2010;4:CD006538.

4. Nussbaum ML, Laskin DM, Best AM. Closed versus open reduction of mandibular condylar fractures in adults: a meta analysis. J Oral Maxillofac Surg 2008;66:1087–92.

5. Singh V, Bhagol A, Goel M, et al. Outcomes of open versus closed treatment of mandibular subcondylar fractures: a prospective randomized study. J Oral Maxillofac Surg 2010;68(6):1304–9.

6. Danda AK, Muthusekhar MR, Narayanan V, et al. Open versus closed treatment of unilateral subcondylar and condylar neck fractures: a prospective, randomized clinical study. J Oral Maxillofac Surg 2010;68(6):1238–41.

7. Villareal PM, Monje F, Junguera LM, et al. Mandibular condyle fractures: determinants of treatment and outcome. J Oral Maxillofac Surg 2004;62(2):155–63.

8. MacArthur CJ, Donald PJ, Knowles J, et al. Open reduction-fixation of mandibular subcondylar fractures. A review. Arch Otolaryngol Head Neck Surg 1993;119(4):403–6.

9. Haug RH, Assael LA. Outcomes of open versus closed treatment of mandibular subcondylar fractures. J Oral Maxillofac Surg 2001;59(4):370–5.

10. Ellis E 3rd, Throckmorton GS. Bite forces after open or closed treatment of mandibular condylar process fractures. J Oral Maxillofac Surg 2001;59(4):389–95.

11. Yang WG, Chen CT, Tsay PK, et al. Functional results of unilateral mandibular condylar process fractures after open and closed treatment. J Trauma 2002; 52(3):498–503.

12. Ellis E 3rd, Simon P, Throckmorton GS. Occlusal results after open or closed treatment of fractures of the mandibular condylar process. J Oral Maxillofac Surg 2000;58(3):260–8.

13. Zachariades N, Mezitis M, Mourouzis C, et al. Fractures of the mandibular condyle: a review of 466 cases. Literature review, reflections on treatment and proposals. J Craniomaxillofac Surg 2006; 34(7):421–32.

14. Vural E, Ragland J, Key JM. Manually provided temporary maxillomandibular fixation in the treatment of selected mandibular fractures. Otolaryngol Head Neck Surg 2008;138:528–30.

REFERENCES (KELLMAN)

1. Wilson IF, Lokeh A, Benjamin CI, et al. Prospective comparison of panoramic tomography (zonography) and helical computed tomography in the diagnosis and operative management of mandibular fractures. Plast Reconstr Surg 2001;107: 1369–75.

2. Lee C, Mankani MH, Kellman RM, et al. Minimally invasive approaches to mandibular fractures. Facial Plast Surg Clin North Am 2001;9: 475–87.

3. Kellman RM. Endoscopically assisted repair of subcondylar fractures of the mandible. Arch Facial Plast Surg 2003;5:244–50.

4. Eckelt U, Schneider M, Erasmus F, et al. Open v. closed treatment of mandibular condylar process– a prospective randomized multi-center study. J Craniomaxillofac Surg 2006;34:306–14.

5. Singh V, Bhagol A, Goel M, et al. Outcomes of open versus closed treatment of mandibular subcondylar fractures: a prospective randomized study. J Oral Maxillofac Surg 2010;68(6):1304–9.

6. Danda AK, Muthusekhar MR, Narayanan V, et al. Open versus closed treatment of unilateral subcondylar and condylar neck fractures: a prospective, randomized clinical study. J Oral Maxillofac Surg 2010;68(6):1238–41.

7. Kellman RM. Maxillofacial Trauma. In: Cummings otolaryngology head and neck surgery. 5th edition. Philadelphia: Mosby; 2010. p. 318–41.

8. Schneider M, Erasmus F, Gerlach KL, et al. Open reduction and internal fixation v. closed treatment and mandibulomaxillary fixation of fractures of the mandible condylar process: a randomized, prospective, multicenter study with special evaluation of fracture level. J Oral Maxillofac Surg 2008;66:2337–44.

9. Kerner CH, Undt G, Rasse M. Surgical reduction and fixation of intracapsular condylar fracture: a follow-up study. Int J Oral Maxillofac Surg 1998;27:191–4.

10. Raveh J, Redli M, Markwalder TM. Operative management of 194 cases of combined maxillofacial-frontobasal fractures: principles and surgical modifications. J Oral Maxillofac Surg 1984;42:555–64.

11. Raveh J. Open reduction of the dislocated fixed condylar process: indications and surgical procedures. J Oral Maxillofac Surg 1989;47:120–6.

12. Mueller RV, Czerwinski M, Lee C, et al. Condylar fracture repair: use of the endoscope to advance traditional treatment philosophy. Facial Plast Surg Clin North Am 2006;14:1–9.

13. Zide MF, Kent JN. Indications for open reduction of mandibular condyle fractures. J Oral Maxillofac Surg 1983;41:89–98.

Facial Reanimation
Discussion and Debate

Kofi Boahene, MD[a],*, Patrick Byrne, MD[b],*,
Barry M. Schaitkin, MD[c],*

KEYWORDS

- Facial reanimation • Facial paralysis • Nonsurgical therapy • End-to-side anastomosis

---

Facial Reanimation Panel Discussion

Kofi Boahene, Patrick Byrne, and Barry M. Schaitkin address questions for discussion and debate:

1. What forms of nonsurgical therapy (physical therapy, electrical stimulation, and so forth) do you recommend to improve the outcome of facial paralysis and why?

2. Explain your preoperative assessment tool for deciding what to do (Eye reanimation? Who needs a medial canthoplasty? and so forth).

3. How do you assess the results of management of facial paralysis?

4. Discuss the use of end-to-side anastomosis (Viterbo concept of something for nothing). Should it be used; why or why not?

5. What is your preferred method for temporalis muscle transposition and why? Are there any tricks to improving the results?

6. Do you use cross-facial nerve jump grafts and use them for free muscle innervation? If so, what are the pearls you have learned from this technique and when do you use it?

7. *Analysis:* Over the past 5 years, how has your approach evolved or what have you learned/observed in working with reanimation?

What forms of nonsurgical therapy (physical therapy, electrical stimulation, and so forth) do you recommend to improve the outcome of facial paralysis and why?

BOAHENE

To date, the best reanimation surgeries have fallen far short of completely restoring the complex expressive movements and function characteristic of the normal unparalyzed face. This is partly because changes in the somatotopic arrangement that occur in the facial nucleus and the facial motor cortex cannot be directly corrected with reanimation surgery. To influence the inaccessible aspects

---

[a] Department of Otolaryngology–Head and Neck Surgery, Johns Hopkins University School of Medicine, Baltimore, MD, USA
[b] Department of Otolaryngology–Head and Neck Surgery, Facial Plastic and Reconstructive Surgery, Johns Hopkins University School of Medicine, Baltimore, MD, USA
[c] Department of Otolaryngology, University of Pittsburgh, Pittsburgh, 5200 Centre Avenue, Suite 211, PA 15232, USA
* Corresponding authors.
E-mail addresses: kofiboah@yahoo.com; pbyrne2@jhmi.edu; schaitkinb@upmc.edu

Facial Plast Surg Clin N Am 20 (2012) 383–402
doi:10.1016/j.fsc.2012.05.006
1064-7406/12/$ – see front matter © 2012 Elsevier Inc. All rights reserved.

of the facial neuromuscular network, nonsurgical therapies are needed. Various forms of nonsurgical therapy and intervention have been shown to minimize the effects of aberrant facial nerve regeneration, improve facial symmetry, help patients adapt a new social smile, and maximize the effectiveness of any reinnervated facial muscle or substitute muscle. Facial neuromuscular retraining, speech therapy, and the selective use of chemodenervation agents are the main nonsurgical interventions I recommend for facial paralysis.

Facial neuromuscular rehabilitation (fNMR) or mime therapy was introduced in 1980 in the Netherlands, specifically for patients with facial nerve paralysis, through collaborative work between mime actors and clinicians. Neuromuscular retraining unlinks undesired motions from desired ones using slow, small-amplitude, desired motions while consciously suppressing the undesired ones. As the undesired activity is suppressed, the range of the primary movement gradually extends, increasing excursion, strength, and motor control. Surface electromyographic (EMG) feedback, mirror feedback, and video biofeedback are essential complementary tools that help bring desired movements to conscious control. Although there is a paucity of well-designed, randomized controlled trials on the effectiveness of facial exercises on the functional outcome of facial paralysis, selected publications support its beneficial role. Pereira and colleagues performed a systematic review and meta-analysis of 132 studies that investigated the role of facial exercises in facial paralysis and concluded that it was effective. Beurskens and Heymans in a randomized controlled trial concluded that mime therapy improved facial symmetry and reduced the severity of facial paralysis.

My facial reanimation patients see a physical therapist before any intervention who specializes in fNMR. I also recommend early facial retraining exercises to Bell palsy patients to minimize the severity of any synkinesis that may occur. A study by Nakamura and colleagues showed that biofeedback works better for prevention of synkinesis as opposed to treatment of synkinesis. Due to the intense efforts needed to achieve visible improvement in their synkinesis, patients often fail to reach their desired goal because of the difficulty of maintaining motivation during training. Initiating biofeedback techniques soon after a facial injury motivates patients to prevent rather than treat synkinesis.

Once patients have become comfortable with their self-directed exercises, I often aid their progress with selective chemodenervation with botulinum toxin injection. The selective use of botulinum toxin helps uncouple facial muscle groups involved in synkinesis. I treat both the paralyzed and unparalyzed face to produce balance and symmetry. Patients with lip incontinence, masticatory difficulties, and articulation changes undergo speech therapy. A speech therapist measures interlabial pressures and provides exercises that aid with lip seal. In selected cases, I use injectable fillers to aid with lip continence.

Facial exercise therapy is also essential in the acquisition and adaption of a temporal smile after a temporalis tendon transfer procedure. The main goal of temporal smile therapy is to transfer upper lip excursion in smile function to the transposed temporalis muscle. There are 3 main phases in the therapy involved in acquiring the temporal smile:

1. The first phase, the mandibular phase, involves mobilizing the mandible to contract the transferred temporalis muscle to elevate the oral commissure.
2. The second phase, the voluntary temporal smile, replaces the mandibular phase and involves contraction of the temporalis muscle without movement of the mandible.
3. The third phase, the spontaneous temporal smile, concentrates on adapting the voluntary temporal smile as the expressive smile for social settings.

Patients with facial paralysis are increasingly inquiring about the role of acupuncture in the treatment of facial paralysis. I do not recommend for or against the adjunctive pursuit of acupuncture but caution my patients from delaying definitive care when nerve grafting is recommended. In addition, I caution my patients concerning the potential for direct nerve injury from the acupuncture needle when repaired nerves are superficial.

BYRNE

I encourage physical therapy. Although functional electrical stimulation has a body of supportive literature for spinal cord injury, I do not believe this is the case for facial rehabilitation. The data for targeted facial retraining via traditional physical therapy—with or without biofeedback—are not conclusive either. There is a logical and neurophysiologic basis, however, for encouraging this.

We work with a physical therapist who has a particular interest in facial retraining. The goals are 2-fold, depending on the nature of the paralysis:

1. The first goal is to encourage purposeful and appropriate movements.
2. An equally important second goal for many (most) patients is to limit synkinesis.

SCHAITKIN

I use physical therapy extensively in the rehabilitation of nonsurgical and surgical patients who have had facial paralysis. I have done so since 1991. Initially I referred patients to Richard Balliet and colleagues.[1] Balliet used the phrase, "neuromuscular retraining of facial paralysis," referring to combining patient education in basic facial anatomy, physiology, and kinesiology; relaxation training; sensory stimulation; EMG biofeedback; voluntary facial exercises with mirror feedback; and spontaneously elicited facial movements.[2] Most recently I have been working with Todd Henklemann,[2] using his physical therapy techniques. I have been impressed with the ability of these techniques to improve scores using the Ross-Fradet grading system.[3] Much of this work owes it origins and proliferation to Jackie Diels.[4] Her concepts of incorporating surface EMG biofeedback with a comprehensive rehabilitation strategy have solid foundation and are used effectively by therapists throughout the country. This is not a single modality approach to facial paralysis patients.

When evaluating these techniques, patients need to be separated into those who have an intact nerve after and are recovering from a viral facial paralysis and those who have had interruption of the nerve and nerve grafting, substitution, or other non-neural reanimation techniques. For the viral facial paralysis patients, I see no need to send patients who are in excellent prognostic groups: incomplete paralysis, excellent evoked electrical testing in the first 10 days, or early onset of recovery after complete paralysis (<4 weeks). I have seen benefits on multiple levels for sending patients who have are not in these groups. Early therapy is aimed at patients who have weakness without synkinesis.

Facial nerve physical therapy is often done in concert with the use of botulinum toxin.[5] The Cochrane Collaboration in 2008 published an article, "Physical Therapy for Bell's Palsy" (Idiopathic Facial Paralysis) (Review).[6] They selected randomized and quasi-randomized controlled studies involving physical therapy. Their conclusion was that a review of available literature involved a wide variety of physical therapy techniques used for treating Bell palsy. They found a "lack of high quality evidence to support the use of these strategies." It is my impression, however, that the use of physical therapy for these patients is not controversial (a statement that may, in and of itself, be controversial). The problem with this review is, that even the selected studies it is based on, begin therapy at a variety of times post-insult, making comparisons difficult. Patients not only benefit from the coaching and emotional support of a therapist, but also have documented recovery.

I find the area of electrical stimulation much more controversial, however. Although there are animal studies that suggest that electrical stimulation may have a positive effect in that it shortens the early stage of recovery after rodent facial nerve crush injury,[7] I have not seen it beneficial in my patient population. The vast majority of patients who are seen in my practice after receiving electrical stimulation seem to follow the natural history of the disease, and those who are at the end of the natural history recovery have not shown improvement with additional electrical stimulation. Referring back to the Cochrane article regarding electrical stimulation, "almost all the outcomes reported failed to show any statistically significant difference between electro-therapy or exercises and conventional or no treatment." Some of the results both in animals and humans have shown worse results in the electrical stimulation group.[8,9]

Facial reanimation patients need physical therapy for the following reasons: their facial paralysis is much longer than in viral patients and extends while they wait for nerve growth to occur; they have emotional needs from a facial nerve and sometimes diagnostic point of view; and their best possible outcome, an House-Brackmann (HB) grade III, in the case of simple nerve repair, is considered a poor outcome from a viral facial paralysis standpoint. Patients with nerve substitutions, such as hypoglossal to facial jump grafts, and those with innervations of free muscle transfers must relearn their smile and they greatly benefit from facial retraining with experts who dedicate their practice to the care of facial paralysis patients. Hadlock and colleagues[9] recently described a mixed group of reanimation patients, 111 of whom were sent for physical therapy. Of these, 83% reported subjective improvement and 97% had objective changes using a grading system.

Explain your preoperative assessment tool for deciding what to do (Eye reanimation? Who needs a medial canthoplasty? and so forth)

BOAHENE

My preoperative assessment tool for facial reanimation focuses on determining and documenting the cause of the paralysis, the reversibility of the paralysis, the functional deficits that are present, and the specific goals of patients seeking reanimation. An accurate and thorough preoperative assessment is essential in selecting appropriate reanimation methods and helps prioritize the intervention.

Determining the cause of facial paralysis

The causes of facial paralysis vary widely but can be categorized into

- Idiopathic facial paralysis (Bell palsy)
- Paralysis resulting from tumors (facial neuroma, acoustic neuroma, geniculate hemangioma, parotid neoplasms, and so forth)
- Developmental or traumatic facial paralysis.

Establishing the cause of the facial paralysis gives essential information about the prognosis and expected course of the paralysis. A thorough history is usually adequate to determine the cause of facial paralysis. Adult patients presenting with long-standing paralysis may not have precise information, however, about the etiology of the paralysis. For example, patients with paralysis secondary to birth trauma or early-childhood infection may confuse their acquired paralysis secondary to birth trauma for a developmental paralysis. When necessary, we obtain a high-resolution MRI and temporal bone CT scan to evaluate the intracranial and extracranial course of the facial nerve and to evaluate for skeletal and soft tissue abnormalities. Even after a thorough history and high-resolution imaging studies, the cause of a facial paralysis may remain elusive and a diagnostic surgical exploration may be necessary. Occult neoplasms can masquerade as Bell palsy, which delays the timely diagnosis and treatment of the neoplasm and the resulting facial paralysis. We obtain and document information about the duration and progression of the paralysis and the functional deficits present and a standardized quality-of-life assessment is obtained.

Establishing if the paralysis is reversible

When evaluating patients for potential facial reanimation, it is important to establish whether the paralysis is reversible or irreversible. The reversibility of the paralysis depends on several factors, including

- Duration
- Degree of injury (complete vs partial)
- Status of the facial muscles and facial nerve.

A reversibly paralyzed facial muscle has physiologically viable muscle fibers with intact neuromuscular junctions that respond to ingrowing axons. Reinnervating such a muscle results in a functional and contracting muscle that can restore tone and movement to the face. On the contrary, atrophic and fibrotic muscles (irreversible paralysis) have both mechanical and physiologic barriers to incoming axons and do not respond to reinnervation. In irreversible facial paralysis, options that rely on recruiting a new source of functional muscle to replace the damaged facial muscles are required for facial reanimation.

The duration of facial paralysis is an approximate predictor of the reversibility of the facial paralysis. The returns on nerve grafting after 1 year of paralysis diminish significantly. When the facial nerve is known to be anatomically continues, nerve grafting after 2 years is possible and has been reported. An EMG is helpful in providing objective support for the reversibility of the facial paralysis. I obtain an EMG on all patients who are considered for facial reinnervation procedures. The presence of persistent electrical silence with attempted voluntary movement on EMG signifies irreversible paralysis and in such patients we consider transfer of regional or free functional muscle. When the EMG reveals fibrillation potentials, then the paralyzed facial muscle is a viable end organ and options for nerve grafting, depending on the duration of paralysis, are considered.

Assessment of functional and aesthetic deficits from facial paralysis

Paralysis of the facial muscles results in functional and aesthetic changes that affect eye protection, breathing, smiling, lip continence, and speech. Compensatory changes on the contralateral unparalyzed side also contribute to the overall morbidity of facial paralysis. Faulty regeneration of repaired or spontaneously recovering nerve may result in sequelae that may be worse than the facial paralysis. In planning for facial reanimation, I assess functional and aesthetic changes by a subunit approach (ie, the upper face [brows and eyelids], midface [smile, lip levators, nasal patency, and lip continence], lower face [lip depressors], and neck [platysma muscle]). In addition, I assess for global facial response to facial paralysis and nerve regeneration, including signs of aberrant reinnervation (ie, hypercontraction, hypokinesis, and synkinesis).

Assessment and reanimation of the upper face

Brow ptosis The ptotic brow resulting after facial paralysis produces heaviness along the temporal brow and may obstruct the peripheral visual field. The visual field obstruction is usually more pronounced in elderly patients. In younger patients, the aesthetic asymmetry from brow ptosis is usually more bothersome than visual field obstruction. Patients are asked to frown and raise their brow to document the dynamic changes in the frontalis muscle. By manually elevating the temporal brow, we determine the degree to which brow ptosis contributes to visual field obstruction and select the best vector for brow pexy if necessary. Endoscopic brow suspension for female patients and younger patients is our main approach to correcting paralytic brow ptosis. In elderly patients who are aesthetically less sensitive, we find the open midforehead or a temporal brow lift satisfactory. The emphasis on brow suspension in the paralyzed forehead is placed on the temporal portion of the brow because that portion tends to droop the most. We use selective chemodenervation of the contralateral frontalis muscle to help achieve forehead and brow symmetry. I personally do not favor the routine use of cross-facial nerve grafting for reanimating the paralyzed brow although it has been successfully demonstrated. This is due to the need for harvesting a sural nerve graft, scarring from exploring both sides of the face, and risk of injury to the intact contralateral facial nerve.

Eyelids Paralysis of the orbicularis oculi muscle is associated with significant dysfunction that can lead to keratitis, corneal abrasion and loss of vision. Restoring eyelid function and corneal protection remains one of the primary focuses of our reanimation efforts in facial paralysis. Our preoperative assessment of the paralyzed eyelid systematically documents the ability of patients to voluntarily and involuntarily blink, corneal sensation, globe position (positive vs negative vector globe), medial and lateral canthal laxity, position of lower lacrimal punctum, tearing, and degree of scleral show. Terzis and Kyere have published a grading system for eyelid paralysis, which we have found helpful. The eyelid examination is documented by video and photographic capture. With the head in a neutral position, voluntary and involuntary blinking is recorded. Patients are then asked to close their eye gently and then tightly. The presence or absence of twitching, spasm, or synkinetic movement of the lips and neck muscles are noted. Patients who are considered for nerve grafting undergo preoperative EMG. We address the upper and lower eyelids separately with either static procedures, regional muscle transfer, or nerve grafting procedures based on patient age, degree of lagophthalmos, ectropion, and EMG findings.

Table 1 shows the indications and various techniques we use in addressing the paralyzed eyelid. In younger patients with reversible paralysis of the orbicularis oculi muscle, we strongly consider reinnervating the muscle with nerve grafts either by direct muscle nerotization or interpositional grafting if the nerve branch to the muscle can be identified. When considering upper eyelid loading, we use the platinum chain implants weighing between 0.8 g and 1.2 g. Heavier weights often result in excessive mechanical ptosis that may obstruct vision and result in an unacceptable eyelid asymmetry. We recommend upper eyelid loading more for its ability to aid in voluntary blinking than for its gravity effects. Patients with a negative vector eyes where the globe is anteriorly positioned are not good candidates for upper eyelid loading. This is because the implant sits over the protruding globe and the resulting inertia makes it less effective in initiating eyelid movement. In patients with thin upper eyelid skin, we recommend placing a barrier over fascia or allograft barrier over the implant to minimize extrusion. The lower eyelid position and function is arguable more important in corneal protection in the upper eyelid. The essential functional features of the lower eyelid are its vertical position, pumping effect on the lacrimal canaliculi, apposition of the lacrimal puncta to the globe, and the medial and lateral canthal support.

Table 1 shows indications and the technique we commonly use to address the paralyzed lower eyelid. As a general principle, we favor dynamic reanimation of the lower eyelid over static procedures. Among the static eyelid procedures

Table 1
(Boahene) Problem-oriented facial reanimation surgery

Anatomic Site	Procedure	Indication
Brow	Unilateral endoscopic brow lift Temporal brow lift	Paralytic brow ptosis, temporal brow hooding, peripheral visual field obstruction from ptotic brow
	Midforehead brow lift	Limited to elderly men with deep forehead rhytids
Upper eyelid	Upper eyelid loading with platinum chain implant. Fascia or allograft barrier is placed over the implant in thin skin eyelids	Poor blink, 2–3 mm lagophthalmos, favorable globe position
	Minitemporalis muscle transfer	Poor corneal sensation, absence Bell phenomenon, poor blink, negative vector globe
	Levator advancement or plication	Blepharoptosis secondary to aberrant facial nerve regeneration
Lower eyelid	Lower eyelid vertical suspension with a spacer graft	Ectropion with >2–3 mm scleral show
	Lower eyelid fascial sling suspension	Ectropion, patient with medial and lateral canthal tendon laxity, lacrimal punctum eversion
	Medial canthopexy. Perform through a postcaruncular incision with canthal supetention to periorbital posterior-to-posterior lacrimal crest	Medial canthal laxity, medial eyelid margin eversion, lacrimal punctum displaced away from globe, lacrimal punctum can be distractly laterally past the medial limbus
	Lateral canthopexy	Lateral canthal laxity, used in combination with medial canthopexy
	Tarsal strip, canthal tightening	Extreme canthal laxity in elderly patients
	Direct neurotization of orbicularis oculi muscle (jump graft from ipsilateral facial nerve stump or hypoglossal nerve)	Presence of fibrillation potential or reduced motor activity on EMG, resected or unidentifiable ipsilateral facial nerve branch to orbicularis, young or middle-aged patient
Upper lip	Direct nerve repair with end-to-end coaptation Interpositional grafting Transposition of intratemporal facial nerve to hypoglossal nerve with end-to-side anatomosis with 30% partial hypoglossal neurotomy Hypoglossal to facial nerve jump grafting Hyoglossal to facial nerve transfer Cross-facial nerve grafting	Lower facial hypokinesis, asymmetry, distorted smile
Lower lip	Direct repair or with cable graft when proximal and distal ends of the marginal nerve branch can be identified	Asymmetric lower lip depression during smile with EMG evidence for a reversible paralysis
		Asymmetric smile with EMG evidence of irreversible paralysis
	Transfer of marginal branch to hypoglossal nerve for end-to-side coaptation	When the proximal facial nerve in unavailable but a long marginal branch reaches the hypoglossal nerve
	Direct neurotization of depressor labia muscle	When distal facial nerve unavailable but facial muscle are viable
	Diagastric tendon transfer	Delayed repair of isolated lower lip paralysis
Neck	Platysma resection	Synkinesis with platysma hyper contraction
	Platysma and SMAS suspension	Correction of paralytic jowling and platysma banding

available, we place more emphasis on procedures that maintain or improve the vertical height of the lower eyelid because loss of tone in the paralyzed orbicularis oculi muscle results in eyelid ectropion. We reserve lid-shortening procedures to elderly patients who have excessive canthal laxity. Although lateral canthal tightening is commonly described, laxity of the medial canthus is often overlooked. Our main indications for medial canthopexy are eversion of the medial lower eyelid margin, distraction of the lacrimal punctum away from the globe, and the ability to distract the lower eyelid lacrimal punctum lateral to the medial limbus (**Fig. 1**). Faulty regeneration of the facial nerve innervating the upper eyelid muscle can result in obstructive blepharospasm that appears as blepharoptosis. This ptosis temporarily

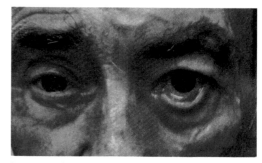

Fig. 1. Paralytic lower eyelid ectropion with eversion of lacrimal puncatum away from globe.

responds for chemodenervation and also to levator aponeurosis advancement for a more long-term correction.

Assessment and reanimation of the paralyzed midface

Dynamic reanimation of the paralyzed midface aims to restore upper lip elevation and midfacial tone and symmetry at rest. In addition, midfacial reanimation has the potential to improve nasal breathing in cases of paralytic nasal obstruction and improve vertical support of the paralyzed lower eyelid. Improving tone in the midface and lip seal also helps with speech and lip incontinence. In assessing the midface for smile restoration, the pattern of smile based on movement on the contralateral side is determined. Specifically, we determine the predominant vector of movement during upper lip excursion. In tendon or muscle transfer procedures, we try to reproduce this movement by inserting the transferred muscle along this vector. Patients are asked to produce a gentle smile followed by an exaggerated full smile while being video recorded. A ruler is position next to the oral commissure of the nonparalyzed side to serve as a scale for measuring the degree of excursion off videos. We also evaluate the function of the masseter and temporalis muscles. When surgical procedures have

previously been performed around the temporalis muscle, a muscle stimulator is useful in determining contraction of the temporalis muscle. We clinically determine and document function of cranial nerves V, IX, and XII as potential motor sources for nerve grafting. Nasal examination is performed to document static and dynamic valve collapse on the paralyzed side. Lip continence and speech assessment are performed by a speech pathologist and measurements of interlabial pressures from the midlips and lateral lips are obtained.

Assessment and reanimation of the lower face

Lower lip The lower lip is essential in sealing the lip for lip continence to prevent drooling and in the generation of plosive sounds during speech. The depressors of the lower lip also contribute to the production of a full smile that reveals both the upper and lower lip. Isolated injury to the marginal branch of the facial nerve is common and manifests in a distorted smile (**Fig. 2**). Lower lip function before reanimation is assessed with video documentation. Patients are asked to smile with a gentle and an exaggerated smile to determine the contribution of the lower lip depressors to their natural smile. Interlabial pressures are

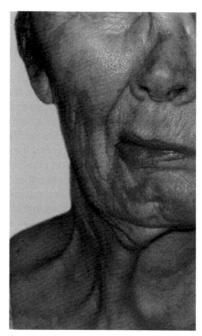

Fig. 2. (Boahene) Lower face paralysis.

measured to objectively document differences between the paralyzed and normal sides of the lip. In patients who have recovered from previous facial paralysis, it is essential to document the presence of synkinetic movement with other facial

muscles as well as the effects of any platysma hypercontracture on lip movement. The degree of lip atrophy is documented to support the need for lip augmentation. **Table 1** shows procedure use for lower lip reanimation.

Neck The changes in the neck after facial paralysis are mainly seen in the platysma muscle and may be negligible or severe. The platysma muscle is often the recipient of excessive innervation after facial nerve injury with spontaneous recovery and after nerve repair. This manifests as hypercontracture of the platysma muscle that produces a tight feeling in the neck. The platsyma muscle extends over the mandible and continues with the submusculoapaneurotic system (SMAS) system of the midface. As a depressor of the lower face, hypercontraction on the platysma muscle is a major antagonist to lip

elevation and can impair movement of the upper lip when smiling. Resection of the hypercontracting platysma muscle or temporary chemodenervation relieves the facial tightness and may allow better excursion of the lip levators. In assessing for platysma resection, patients are asked to smile broadly and presence and location of tight platysma band are marked. The excursion of the oral commissure is recorded on video before and after division of the platysma muscles. We commonly perform platysma muscle resection under local anesthesia through small 1-cm incisions.

BYRNE

This is a lengthy process for me. An initial new patient consult is routinely scheduled for 1 hour—and we use that time up. We discuss the functional aspects of their facial nerve disorder (most importantly, eye protection, but also often speech, oral competence, and nasal breathing) as well as the psychosocial aspects. The psychosocial impact of the facial paralysis is more important to most patients. I believe that we have an obligation during the preoperative assessment to educate patients about symmetry and how faces are perceived by observers. It is a complex topic, but the patients who comprehend this find that it reli is empowering.

To grossly simplify, the social aspect of facial paralysis is a problem of perceived asymmetry; because all faces have some degree of asymmetry, observers routinely ignore this in daily life. With facial paralysis, suddenly the degree of asymmetry is such that it triggers conscious recognition on the part of the observer. Thus, the reality is that the problem is not the dysfunction but the degree of asymmetry that is produced and whether or not this is enough for others to routinely notice. This is our great opportunity for helping patients. We analyze the entire face—upper third, middle third, and lower third—and systematically seek ways to improve 2 things: (1) symmetry) and (2) attractiveness. These are inextricably linked.

As for specific decisions, there are a few personal preferences. I engage patients in personal banter early in the consultation and try to elicit laughter, observing all the while their own particular adaptive and maladaptive facial movement patterns. I believe that for most patients

with brow asymmetry significant enough to warrant intervention, a bilateral endoscopic brow lift is the best choice. There are exceptions. Not all patients need anything done to their lids. Many need nothing surgical. A simple rule to assess risk of exposure keratopathy that I heard years ago from Dr Seiff at UCSF is using the acronym, BAD:

> B = Bell phenomemen—those without are at greater risk
>
> A = Anesthesia of the cornea—also a greater risk patient
>
> D = Dry eye history

Many patients benefit from upper lid loading, and we prefer the platinum chain (**Fig. 3**). (For the lower lid, if lateral ectropion is present [particularly, if symptomatically relieved by the application of gentle digital pressure supporting the lower lid, mimicking a canthopexy], then I usually prefer the lateral transorbital canthopexy, as described by Kris Moe and colleagues[10] [**Fig. 4**]). This is a procedure that is reversible, adjustable, and preserves native anatomy well without shortening the horizontal aperture. It is not ideal for older patients in whom the horizontal dimension of the lid is expanded, however. Those patients tend to require horizontal shortening, such as with a tarsal strip procedure. Medial ectropion requires a specific medial canthopexy. Lid retraction is treated when clinically significant. This is a tough problem, particularly in patients with a negative vector (**Fig. 5**).

The decision-making process for midfacial and lower facial reanimation is individually determined.

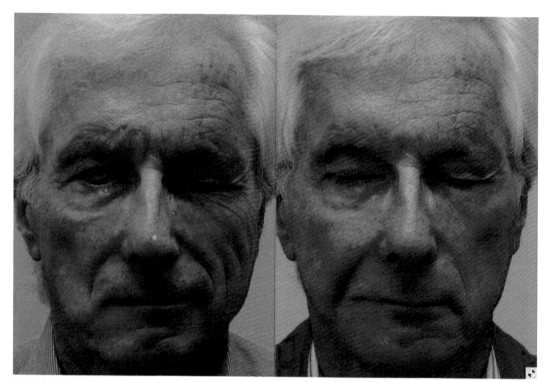

Fig. 3. (Byrne) Paralytic lagoothalmos treated with platinum chain loading to left upper eyelid.

Certainly if the paralysis is caught early we typically offer reinnervation techniques. If it is of long-standing duration, then reanimation via either free tissue transfer or regional muscle transfer is the treatment of choice.

SCHAITKIN

When faced with a patient requiring facial reanimation, I begin with the following historical data[11]:

- What was the cause of the facial paralysis?
- Is the paralysis complete?
- How long has the paralysis been present?

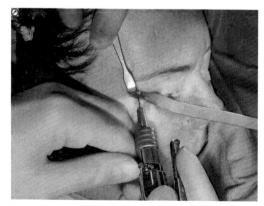

Fig. 4. (Byrne) Lateral transorbital canthopexy. Kris Moe described this useful technique. It is a powerful procedure that preserves anatomy and is reversible, does not shorten the horizontal aperture, avoids a lateral canthotomy, and is easy to perform.

- How old is the patient?
- Is the patient in good health?
- What is the patient's psychological status; in particular, what are the patient's expectations and are they realistic?
- What is the patient's life expectancy?
- Are there other cranial nerves involved? Pay attention, especially, to the trigeminal, vagus, and hypoglossal.
- Which surgical procedures have already been performed?

I then select from the range of dynamic and static procedures based on the answers to these questions and the realistic expectations of the patient. For the eye, I consider particularly if any neural intervention can be expected at some point. This influences not only the reanimation technique but also the expectation of skin tone and lower lid placement. Restricting myself to just the eye for this question, I think it is best to assume that this is a patient who is not expecting any neural intervention but is being reanimated in the absence of nerve continuity. Starting from superior to inferior, I evaluate for the presence of brow ptosis.

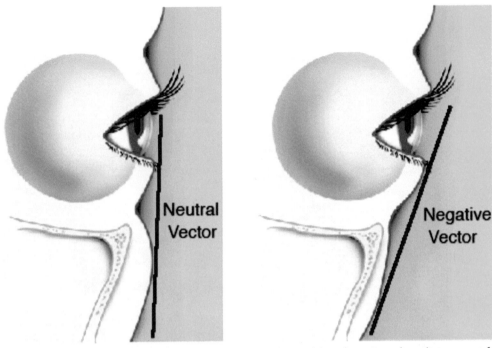

Fig. 5. (Byrne) Illustration demonstrating the negative vector. Patients with such anatomy have less support for the anterior lamella. The lower lid retraction that develops with facial paralysis is difficult to treat, requiring lower lid slings, spacer grafts, and/or midface lifts. Importantly, these patients are not well served by lower lid shortening procedures, such as the tarsal strip tarshorrhaphy.

I frequently accept some element of brow ptosis to enable excellent eye protection and re-animation. My tendency is to use an upper eyelid gold weight implant for patients who do not have a widely open eye at rest and who have an office gold weight assessment that does not show significant ptosis with the gold weight taped to the mid-upper eyelid (5 mm above the lash line). For those who do have significant ptosis, I use a palpebral eyelid spring.[12,13]

The lower eyelid I generally manage with a lower eyelid shortening procedure in patients who have lax skin, particularly older patients. Younger patients I manage with a subcilliary or transconjunctival lid augmentation procedure with either alloderm or conchal cartilage.

I think the most controversial aspect is what to do with the medial canthal region. Medial paralytic ectropian repair, although it may not be controversial, is more difficult than the other aspects of repair.

For planning, I have been impressed with the staging system algorithm for lower eyelid reanimation as proposed by Moe and Kao[10] and I think it is important that practitioners be familiar with the ectropion grading scale. As part of evaluating the eye, of course, the entire eye has to be examined both supine and seated. Particularly when faced with lower eyelid issues, I am documenting the patient's snap test as well as the position of the lower lid relative to the limbus. In addition, I look at the position of the lacrimal punctum. In elderly patients, I am more inclined to perform a medial canthal plication or canthoplasty. I have not been performing the more elegant medial canthal reconstruction, which requires a precaruncular exposure. I think this is certainly an area of controversy and will be interested in the other authors' experiences with reconstructing the medial canthus.

When reconstructing the smile, I again take the questions at the beginning to heart, particularly when deciding if a patient is likely to enjoy the results of procedures that may take more than a year to begin to function. The lower face and the eye are always reanimated separately. The planning is based on the work of Leonard Rubin[14] describing the muscles and vectors of the basic smile types.

How do you assess the results of management of facial paralysis?

BOAHENE

Currently, there is no single assessment tool or grading scale that adequately captures the outcomes of facial reanimation surgery. Proper documentation and secondary analysis of outcomes data are essential in objectively evaluating and reporting the effectiveness of our reanimation protocols. For documenting and analyzing outcomes, video capture of dynamic facial movement provides more useful information than static photographs. Hence, all patients who undergo a facial reanimation procedure receive a standard pretreatment and post-treatment video assessment.

- First, patients are asked to talk while being video recorded, allowing documentation of their involuntary facial movements.
- The patients are then asked to repetitively blink, raise their brows, close their eye gently and then tightly, smile softly and then broadly, purse their lips, and then grimace. These voluntary facial movements are video recorded.
- In select cases, EMG evaluation of reinnervated muscles is obtained.
- Patients who undergo smile restoration or lip procedures are also seen by a speech therapist for a speech assessment and measurement of interlabial pressure.
- Analysis for facial symmetry, eyelid function, and lip excursion are secondarily obtained from the videos and photos.
- Patients are then interviewed to document their functional status regarding visual obstruction, eye protection, nasal breathing, smile in controlled and social settings, lip continence, and facial tightness or discomfort.
- Patients are then asked to complete a quality-of-life assessment tool.

BYRNE

We take standardized photographs with the full range of facial movements. We capture standardized video recordings preoperatively and post-operatively. We then have the results graded by independent observers as well as recording patient self-assessments.

SCHAITKIN

There are many systems available for evaluating facial function using a variety of tools. A controversial point is that they are all lacking in their ability to translate the results fully.[15]

The American Academy of Otolaryngology–Head and Neck Surgery (AAO-HNS) recognizes the HB system. This universal, easily applied system was designed for recovery from Bell palsy. It assumes an intact nerve with recovery and is based heavily on synkinesis. With nerve grafts, as an example, the best one can do is an HB grade III. So, all patients achieve an HB grade III, IV, or V if the procedure had any impact, making comparison of techniques and results difficult. Video systems and photographic systems have been used extensively as well.[15] The facial nerve committee of the AAO-HNS, as one of its last official bits of business before being dissolved, tried to make the HB system available for more reanimation techniques, but it has not been found to date to add anything to the original system.[16]

The Ross-Fradet system allows for patients to be scored over a broader range and, therefore, separates them, allowing patients to have more adequately documented progression if they improve over time. This is useful in reanimation as well as during physical therapy. The Ross-Fradet system separates the face into segments and grades degree of excursion as well as resting symmetry and synkinesis. These features make it my current grading system of choice, allowing for easy communication between my physical therapy colleagues and me.[17]

It should be recalled that the grade achieved with these symptoms does not have to improve over time. For example, using the HB system, I have seen patients develop more severe synkinesis over time and go from a grade III to a grade IV.

Discuss the use of end-to-side anastomosis (Viterbo concept of something for nothing). Should it be used; why or why not?

BOAHENE

The end-to-side nerve anastomosis involves grafting the distal end of a transected nerve to the side of a donor nerve without strictly exposing cut ends of axons within the donor nerve. In practice, the end-to-side anastomosis is done with or without an epineural window. The technique of end-to-side nerve coaptation was described more than a century ago but was reintroduced by Viterbo and colleagues in 1992. The merits and potential advantages of the end-to-side nerve anastomosis are clear: a donor nerve can be a source of reinnervating axons without significant morbidity to the donor nerve. The potential clinical implication for facial paralysis is enormous. For example, patients with facial paralysis could undergo early cross-facial nerve grafting using end-to-side anatomosis on the unparalyzed side without much worry about function deficit from the donor nerve. Significant controversy surrounds the concept of end-to-side nerve grafting.

The main point of argument is that there is no true de novo sprouting of axons from a donor nerve (collateral sprouting) without some degree of injury (regenerative sprouting) (ie, intentional or unintentional). True collateral sprouting implies de novo axonal regeneration without nerve injury, which in myelinated nerves is believed to arise from the nodes of Ranvier. Alternatively, the ability of an injured nerve to regenerate by sprouting axons is well established and supported by vast clinical experience from end-to-end nerve coaptation as well as spontaneous nerve recovery after crush injuries.

Several animal studies and a handful of clinical reports have been published on the feasibility of the end-to-side nerve grafting technique. An exhaustive review of this literature by Dvali and Myckatyn in 2008 led to their conclusion that the degree of motor nerve sprouting after end-to-side grafting was dependent on the degree of the motor nerve injury. In view of this, when critical motor axon regeneration is needed, the more reliable end-to-end anastomosis or end-to-side with a clear intentional partial axotomy in the donor nerve is preferable. In spite of this conclusion, true end-to-side coaptation of nerves remains an attractive concept. Yamamoto[18] have separately published their experience with this technique in improving the outcome in partial facial paralysis.

I have discussed the concept of true end-to-side nerve coaptation with several peripheral nerve experts who focus on brachial nerve injuries. These experts each have clinic cases that support the effectiveness of the end-to-side coaptation but they caution against the routine reliance on this approach. I have found the reverse use of the end-to-side nerve coaptation through an epineural window desirable in functionally upgrading (super-charge concept) a partially recovered facial nerve. When the facial nerve partially recovers after an injury, improving the degree of recovery without disrupting the intact nerve fibers is desirable. To preserve the recipient nerve from losing recovered axons, the donor nerve is grafted through an epineural window in an end-to-side fashion. When the donor nerve is the hypoglossal, there is dual innervation of the facial muscle by both the hypoglossal and facial nerves. Clinically, I have observed improved tone, more facial symmetry, and a better-defined melolabial crease. Yamamoto[18] provides more convincing EMG data that support the presence of upgraded innervations.

BYRNE

This strategy has not gained widespread acceptance since its introduction. I do not believe there are many clinical scenarios in which it would be useful. Cross-facial nerve grafts in theory could be performed without damage to the donor nerve. With these procedures, however, I typically want to choose a targeted nerve—such as a buccal branch, which innervates the zygomaticus—and specifically link that to the corresponding branch on the other side. In this scenario, it has been observed that many that donor nerve transection produces little discernible weakness and that some weakening of the contralateral side actually aids in improving symmetry. Likewise, it is well established in the literature that partial transection of the hypoglossal nerve is well tolerated without tongue dysfunction.

The one related application we have been exploring is the use of a cable graft from a partially transected hypoglossal nerve to an epineural window in an intact but only partially recovered facial nerve. This "supercharging" concept has little supportive literature at present and remains somewhat speculative.

SCHAITKIN

I think the entire concept should be considered controversial. I remember being interested in this topic when Dr Viterbo presented it at the University of Pittsburgh in 1993. Since then there has been continued interest. In 1992, Viterbo and colleagues[19] published rat studies, which demonstrated neural sprouting from an end-to-side nerve graft with or without an epineurial window. Sundine used dog facial nerves and compared end-to-end grafts with end-to-side grafts and found them functionally similar.[20] Frey and colleagues[20] performed sural nerve cross-face grafts to stable long-standing paralysis in 7 patients end to side and found that 3 of 3 with long-term follow-up had improvement.[21]

Brenner and colleagues[21] reviewed the end-to-side literature and wrote, "Our interpretation of the [end-to-side] literature suggests that sensory axons may sprout without deliberately attempting to injure them, while motor axons regenerate only in response to a deliberate injury. Experimental and clinical experience with [end-to-side] neurorrhaphy has rendered mixed results. Our interpretation of the literature suggests that the success of this technique is dependent upon axonal injury of motor and possibly sensory nerves."[22]

Clinical experience with end-to-side procedure has been limited and rarely has it been done in the absence of any other reanimation procedure. These small series, although promising, are difficult to interpret because of the overlay of other techniques. The end-to-side, something for nothing procedure, is a surgically appealing prospect for patients with poor recovery after a variety of insults and remains an attractive possibility for the reanimation surgeon.

What is your preferred method for temporalis muscle transposition and why? Are there any tricks to improving the results?

BOAHENE

The temporalis muscle is a fan-shaped muscle that originates from the temporal fossa and inserts on the coronoid process. The temporalis muscle is innervated by the trigeminal nerve and functions in the opening of the mandible. The midsection of the temporalis muscle has traditionally been transposed over the zygomatic arch to the oral commissure to support the paralyzed upper lip. This method of temporalis muscle transfer has several drawbacks. The transposed muscle is expected to contract along an unnatural fiber orientation. It requires sectioning of the muscle belly, harnesses only part of the contractile force of the temporalis muscle, risks disruption of the muscle innervation, and leaves a bulge over the zygomatic arch, which can exaggerate facial asymmetry. I prefer to transfer the temporalis muscle tendon to the modiolus for dynamic reanimation of the paralyzed lip. Transfer of the temporalis tendon instead of a segment of the muscle leaves the muscle tendon unit in its natural orthodromic orientation. The muscle fibers are not disrupted and its innervation is preserved. The procedure can be performed without an external scalp incision. In addition, there is no bulge left over the zygomatic arch as is typical when the muscle is transposed. Transfer of the temporalis tendon instead of the muscle belly avoids muscle fiber injury, keeps the nerve to the muscle undisrupted, and harnesses the force of the entire muscle. The tendon is detached from the lateral and medial aspect of the coronoid process and advanced to the modiolus. The coronoid process is approached directly either through a melolabial fold incision or transoral exposure.

Pearls from Boahene for temporalis muscle transposition:

1. Select the location for inserting the transposed tendon based on the pattern of contraction of the normal lip levators.
2. The majority of the temporalis tendon inserts on the medial aspect of the coronoid process and extends inferiorly toward the buccinator line. Dissecting the tendon to its inferior extend increases the length of the tendon that can be mobilized.
3. Inserting the tendon at its passive length prevents over-retraction of the oral commissure while maintaining the dynamic range of the muscle. Excessively stretching the tendon minimizes the dynamic potential of the transposed muscle.
4. If the tendon cannot reach the modiolus without excessive stretch, a tendon extender (fascia lata, donor tendon) should be used. Alternatively, the muscle may be released from it origin and allowed to slide inferiorly. The temporalis muscle can be released from its origin through a small scalp incision with the aid of an endoscope.
5. Intraoperative stimulation of the temporalis muscle helps determine the ideal tension at which to fixate the tendon.
6. Patients should actively learn to acquire the temporal smile, using the transposed temporalis muscle. Physical therapy started before the procedure helps with the postprocedure therapy.

BYRNE

I started doing all of my cases of temporalis transposition in an orthodromic fashion in 2001. I had previously been trained to use the classic technique using the belly of the muscle origin, and it was my impression that this was the standard technique throughout the United States. Pretty early, it seemed to me, however, on that the functional results were as good when the insertion of the temporalis (we called it a *temporalis tendon transfer* or *T3*, for that reason) was used instead.[23] This prevented the creation of any asymmetry overlying the zygomatic arch and in the temple (**Fig. 6**). There is no surgically created asymmetry. He has no depression in the temple and no fullness overlying the arch. We attempt to optimize the symmetry of the facial morphology. Of the available reanimation techniques that involve muscle transfer, we believe our T3 procedure is optimal to accomplish this. Ultimately, we realized that the procedure could be easily performed via a simple, single incision in the oral cavity or melolabial fold. Since our first publication of our experience with this technique in 2007, it is my impression that it has become the technique of choice at many centers in the United States.

We continually seek ways to improve the results. There are many little steps that help to get a better outcome.

Pearls from Byrne for temporalis transfer:

- Intraoperative stimulation is important to assess the ideal tension on the insertion.

- Preservation of the tendon and surrounding periosteum creates a more robust connection.
- Attaching the tendon via an extension (typically fascia lata for me) across the midline to the contralateral side in cases where there is significant pull of the philtrum away from the paralyzed side prevents an odd stretch of the commissure and improves postoperative symmetry.
- A careful preoperative assessment of patients' contralateral anatomy assists with a symmetric result.
- Persistent physical therapy to retrain into a symmetric smile is as important as anything.
- Very careful attention should be paid to the manner in which the tissue is sutured to the upper and lower lip as well as the modiolus. It must be aesthetically acceptable and with a tight and competent commissure.
- As with all facial reanimation procedures, we explore opportunities to make the face more attractive. This means, frequently, the concomitant performance of purely cosmetic procedure. We have been pleased with these results for many years at our institution (**Fig. 7**).

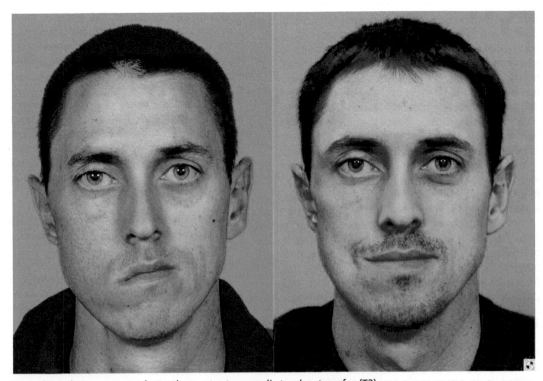

Fig. 6. (Byrne) Young man who underwent a temporalis tendon transfer (T3).

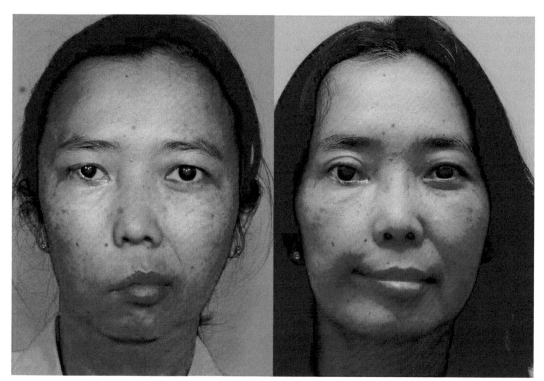

Fig. 7. (Byrne) Temporalis tendon transfer, reversal of tarsorrhaphy, bilateral endoscopic browlift, and chin augmentation.

SCHAITKIN

The history of temporalis transfer is interesting. It was initially described more than 100 years ago. Gillies[24] described transposing the muscle over the zygomatic arch in the 1930s; some investigators have used the entire muscle, and fascial extensions have been used. McLaughlin[25] (1952) described using the muscle leaving it in situ. He described osteotomy of the coranoid process and fascial extensions.[22] The transposed muscle, however, was almost exclusively used for several decades from the 1960s to the 1990s.

The current use of the temporalis by numerous investigators at various institutions seems exclusively to be back to a McLaughlin orthodromic temporalis muscle technique. This minimizes the dissection, has no chance of denervation, eliminates the temporal defect and zygomatic bulge, and allows for the use of the entire muscle for contraction not just a rotated fraction.[26,27]

I do not think much controversy exists here. The nuances of improvement of technique might include the ability to prevent dehiscence of the temporalis attachment to the modiolus in long-standing paralysis and atrophy because little tissue remains for attachment. Hadlock and colleagues[27] describe suture and fascia techniques for augmenting the post-temporalis patient in some cases.

Do you use cross-facial nerve jump grafts and use them for free muscle innervation? If so, what are the pearls you have learned from this technique and when do you use it?

BOAHENE

The facial nerve has approximately 7000 motor axons, which distribute through the terminal branches of the facial nerve to innervate the muscles of facial animation. Because of the collateralization and cross-talk between the facial nerve branches, a terminal branch of the facial nerve on the unparalyzed face can be sacrificed and used as a source of regenerating axons to reinnervate the corresponding muscle group on the paralyzed side through a cross-facial graft. It has clearly been shown through histologic sections that the axonal load from a donor nerve influences the number of axons reaching the distal end of a grafted nerve. Terzis and Kyere showed that axonal loads greater than 900 were needed to achieve excellent facial improvement after cross-facial nerve grafting. This means, at least 13% (900/7000) of the overall facial motor axons are needed to survive the journey through a cross-facial nerve graft to achieve a significant improvement. In view of this, it is clear that more than one small terminal facial branch needs to be sacrificed in cross-facial nerve grafting to achieve a predictable improvement, all other factors been ideal. Sacrificing multiple terminal branches of the nerve will result in a visible weakness in the normal face, which may or may not be desirable. As such cross-facial nerves should be performed with much thought and understanding of its limitations, potential and risks.

My indications for cross-facial nerve grafting are

1. Source of dual innervation in combination with ipsilateral hypoglossal to facial nerve grafting. In this combination, I depend on the hypoglossal

nerve for early reiinervation and restoration of tone. I rely on the cross-facial axons for coordinated facial movement driven by a single facial nucleus.
2. Functional upgrading of a partial or incomplete recovered facial paralysis using the end-to side anastomosis.
3. Dual-source innervation in free functional muscle transfer.

Pearls from Boahene for cross-facial nerve grafting:

1. Observe the smile pattern of the patient and identify the dominant lip elevator muscle. Using a nerve stimulator, identify the nerve fiber that strongly reproduces this smile pattern and avoid sacrificing that nerve branch.
2. Avoid sacrificing 2 adjacent terminal nerve branches
3. Protect the nerve anastomosis with a nerve wrap to minimize escape of axons
4. Clearly mark and document where you leave the distal end of the cross-facial nerve graft for easy identification during the second procedure.

BYRNE

Yes. We use cross-face nerve grafts occasionally in cases of complete paralysis with a known proximal injury, when we are able to intervene early. Often this is performed along with a facial-hypoglossal "babysitter" nerve graft, as described by Terzis and Kyere. I have seen improved tone and some volitional movement, but these results are inconsistent. Cross-face nerve grafts alone for facial paralysis often produce disappointing results, however. We also use them as part of a 2-stage procedure for gracilis muscle innervation.

We have found that results are improved when larger donor nerves are used—thus, providing a higher number of axons for reinnervation. I credit Tessa Hadlock and Mack Chaney with encouraging me to use a much bigger donor facial nerve branch for the first stage cross-face graft procedure. It is a large buccal branch that is taken, that clearly elevates the oral commissure on stimulation. This seems to be key, and the donor site morbidity has been surprisingly minimal.

SCHAITKIN

The initial patient assessment includes diagnosis, prognosis, and other cranial nerve deficits, as discussed in response to question 1, "Explain your preoperative assessment tool for deciding what to do (Eye reanimation? Who needs a medial canthoplasty? and so forth). For patients with an isolated unilateral facial paralysis of long standing (longer than 2 years), I discuss many options, including the use of innervated microvascular transfer. Primarily, my experience is with the use of the gracilis muscle. I have done a 2-stage cross-face graft using endoscopically harvested sural nerve, and I have used a 1-stage jump graft innervation from the hypoglossal. I have had better

success in terms of power with the jump graft, but it requires more training and for older patients only gives a volitional smile. Younger patients sometimes just seem to smile without thinking about tongue movement, but this is not universal, even after physical therapy. The majority of younger patients usually opt for a 2-stage cross-face graft, and older patients often prefer a 1-stage jump graft.

It is not really possible to get a spontaneous, flash, mimetic smile with these techniques. This type of smile, that is a reflex when you see someone you know or hear something funny. Not able to achieved with any of these innervated microvascular procedures, but a camera smile, a volitional smile, is achievable. I do these procedures in partnership with a plastic microvascular surgeon.

In terms of tricks for a jump graft I have learned over the years,

- When transecting the facial nerve at the main trunk, leave the epineurium intact on the posterior aspect of the nerve. This prevents the distal nerve from retracting into the gland.
- Two to three sutures are all that is necessary to hold the nerve together in the parotid.
- The hypoglossal nerve should be used distal to the ansa cervicalis take-off.

- The hypoglossal jump graft should be a lateral divot or cookie bite, and the surgeon should resist the temptation to retrograde dissect the nerve, which only worsens the results.
- A 6-0 nylon suture placed in the midpoint of the hypoglossal nerve before initiating the jump graft divot prevents unintentional overly aggressive depth of the transaction.
- The divot need only be large enough to accept the donor nerve size.
- A Penrose drain placed deep to cranial nerve XII can be stretched by a self-retaining retractor and gently elevate XII into the surgical field and out of the possible pool of blood, facilitating microscopic repair.

Analysis: Over the past 5 years, how has your approach evolved or what have you learned/observed in working with reanimation?

BOAHENE

Restoring balance and movement to the paralyzed face is one of the most rewarding procedures I perform in my practice. Patients with facial paralysis are negatively affected by the fear of permanent facial distortion. Thoroughly explaining the broad options available for reanimating the face gives patients hope and allows them to become active participants in their recovery. A holistic approach to facial paralysis with attention to both the paralyzed and nonparalyzed face yields more satisfying results. The major change in my practice over the past 5 years is the move to intervene sooner with nerve grafting techniques.

In our review of 281 patients with an anatomically intact facial nerve after acoustic neuroma resection, we found that the rate of recovery during the first year could be used to predict long-term outcomes. Whereas in the past I would have waited a year for spontaneous recovery in this patient group, I now attempt to predict long-term outcome by 6 months and intervene by 9 months. I have had great success restoring tone, symmetry, and dynamic movement by transposing the vertical segment of the facial nerve to the hypoglossal nerve. In almost all cases, there has been no significant tongue atrophy or dysfunction. I have observed, however, that although younger patients do well and are able to adapt to smiling with the hypoglossal nerve, older patients

need more prompting to do so. I now routinely combine the cross-facial nerve grafting with the facial to hypoglossal transposition procedure to allow coordinated movement between the 2 sides of the face. In these cases, I only sacrifice a single branch of the normal facial nerve for cross-facial grafting because I depend more on the hyoplossal nerve for tone.

Reanimating the paralyzed eyelids remains my biggest challenge and the most common reason for revision surgery. I have increasingly depended less on heavy upper eyelid loading and more on vertical lower lid suspension for corneal protection. Reinnervating the eyelids muscle has proved superior to static suspension procedures even when the reinnervation was by direct muscle neurotization. Over time, patients are persistently bordered by the effects of synkinesis and facial tightness. Eliminating depressor function of the platysma muscle minimizes complains of facial tightness and allows the lip to elevators to work better. I tend to redirect the cervical branch of the facial nerve toward as the lower lip depressors and routinely section out a segment of the playsma to minimize its contribution to facial tightness. Neuromuscular retraining established early in the process is helpful in dealing with the sequelae of faulty facial nerve regeneration.

BYRNE

A major shift for me has been an unrelenting emphasis on improving facial appearance. This means that the entire face is evaluated for opportunities for

improvement. These patients want to look better. I find that I am discussing more procedures than ever before—bilateral brow lifts, blepharoplasties, facelifting techniques, autologous fat grafting, skin rejuvenation, and so forth, with many if not most patients. I cannot overstate how much this approach has benefitted our patients, more than has a focus simply on the paralysis and asymmetry.

The other change that continues is a preference for early intervention. It has been our observation after acoustic neuroma resections, for example, that if a patient has complete paralysis postoperatively, the timing of recovery is important to assess the likelihood of functionally acceptable regeneration. I believe it unlikely, if no return has begun in the first few months, that the patient will ever regain enough function to be acceptable. Thus, I prefer not to wait a year and instead consider early reinnervation strategies.

There is a threshold for the conscious detection of asymmetry, and this is thus a game of millimeters. I fight for every millimeter.

SCHAITKIN

Over time I have learned to be conservative and respectful of patient expectations. Patients with facial paralysis are devastated. They need someone to tell them that it will never be the way it was and then to sit back and let them absorb that statement and react.

I am more likely to encourage physical therapy. I use Botox more often, especially to the normal side to decrease the asymmetry, which catches the eye of the observer.

Five years more of experience allows me to show them more results of previous/similar problems. It allows me to show my best and worst results to them and allows me to no longer fear or fret if they decide not to have facial reanimation because of what I show them.

Although usually patients and I have no trouble agreeing on a great result, I might think someone has a good result, and the patient may not always think so. This happens most frequently with non-neural techniques, including gold weights, brow lifts, and static suspensions.

I think I now do a better job at providing patients with a range of options and helping them understand the benefits and risks of each.

KOFI BOAHENE OFFERS INSIGHTS OR PERSPECTIVES INTO FACIAL PARALYSIS

Facial animation is an essential part of human communication and is one of our main means of expressing emotions, indexing our physiologic state, and providing nonverbal cues. The loss of this important human quality due to facial paralysis can be devastating and is often associated with depression and social isolation and has an adverse impact on quality of life. In addition, facial paralysis significantly impairs functional eyelid closure, nasal breathing, lip competence, and speech. The goals of facial reanimation are to correct these impaired functional deficits and restore facial symmetry at rest and in animation. The causes of facial paralysis vary broadly and include developmental abnormalities, early childhood infection, vascular compression, inflammatory processes, primary and secondary neoplasms, iatrogenic injuries, trauma, and idiopathic paralysis. Common to these causes of facial paralysis is an interruption at some level along the neuromuscular pathway from the facial motor cortex to the facial muscles. Regardless of the cause of the paralysis, dynamic facial reanimation requires restoration of the nerve muscle network either by nerve and muscle repair or substitution or by a combination of both. Advanced understanding of nerve injury, nerve regeneration, and muscle physiology forms the basis of contemporary approaches to facial reanimation. In this forum, I summarize my personal approach to facial reanimation based on close observation of my patients and from the experiences I have adopted from other experts.

THE FACE WITH FACIAL NERVE IMPAIRMENT

The chronic sequelae of facial paralysis can be described by a continuum of symptoms that ranges from chronic hypokinesis and hypotonus to chronic hypekinesis and hypertonus. Clinically, chronic hypokinesis manifests as brow ptosis, lagopthalmos, ectropion, asymmetric smile, nasal obstruction, lip incontinence, and masticatory and articulatory difficulties. Clinical evidence of chronic hyperkinesis include blepharospasm, mid-facial hypercontracture, muscle spasm, facial tightness, synkinesis, facial tightness, and pain. The approach I select to address these sequelae of facial paralysis and to reanimate the face includes nonsurgical therapy, semi-invasive injectional therapy, and invasive surgical reanimation procedures. Several fundamental tenets guide my approach to reanimation of the paralyzed face.

1. Dynamic reanimation is functionally and aesthetically superior to static suspension.

2. The timing of repair is the most important factor in determining the degree of recovery. I therefore try to intervene at the earliest possible time.

3. All significantly injured nerves regenerate after repair with some degree of aberrancy (synkinesis, hypercontracture, and twitching).

4. More is not always better. More regeneration may result in more aberrancy that may be undesirable and worse than the original paralysis.

5. The paralyzed face is best driven by the ipsilateral facial nucleus.

6. Reinnervating the ipsilateral facial muscles, when feasible, is preferable to transposing substitute muscles.

7. First do no harm. Avoid complete injury of a normally functioning nerve in an attempt to restore movement to the paralyzed face when the outcome is unpredictable. In this respect, I favor partial neurectomy of a donor hypoglossal nerve to complete sacrifice of the hypoglossal nerve.

8. With respect to facial nerve repair, direct repair > interpositional grafting > cranial nerve substitution > cross-facial grafting > direct muscle neurotization.

9. A single anastomosis is preferable to a double anastomosis. Thus, transposing the facial nerve to the hypoglossal nerve is preferable to interpositional grafting between the hypoglossal nerve and the facial nerve.

10. A facial nerve–driven functional muscle transfer produces more volutional movement compared with regional muscle tendon unit transfer.

11. Dynamic reanimation of the eyelids is preferred to static suspension.

12. Neuromuscular retraining is essential for success.

13. Treating the unparalyzed side of the face is as important as treating the paralyzed side.

RECOMMENDED READINGS (BOAHENE)

Pereira L, Obara K, Menacho M, et al. Facial exercise therapy for facial palsy: systematic review and meta-analysis. Clin Rehabil 2011;25(7):649–58.

Beurskens CH, Heymans PG. Mime therapy improves facial symmetry in peple with long-term facial nerve paresis: a randomized controlled trial. Aust J Physiother 2006;52(3):177–83.

Lambert-Prou MP. The temporal smile. Speech therapy for palsy patients after temporal lengthening myoplasty. Rev Stomatol Chir Maxillofac 2003;104(5):274–80.

Dvali LY, Myckatyn TM. End-to-side nerve repair: review of the literature and clinical indications. Hand Clin 2008;24(4):455–60.

Bratzlavsky M, Eecken H. Altered synaptic organization in facial nucleus following facial nerve regeneration: an electrophysiologic study in man. Ann Neurol 1977;2:71–3.

Nakamura K, Toda N, Sakamaki K, et al. Biofeedback rehabilitation for prevention of synkinesis after facial palsy. Otolaryngol Head Neck Surg 2003;128(4):539–43.

Boahene DO, Olsen KD, Driscoll C, et al. Facial nerve paralysis secondary to occult malignant neoplasms. Otolaryngol Head Neck Surg 2004;130(4):459–65.

Rivas A, Boahene KD, Bravo HC, et al. A model for early prediction of facial nerve recovery after vestibular schwannoma surgery. Otol Neurotol 2011;32(5):826–33.

Terzis JK, Kyere SA. Minitendon graft transfer for suspension of the paralyzed lower eyelid: our experience. Plast Reconstr Surg 2008;121(4):1206–16.

SCHAITKIN REFERENCES: NONSURGICAL THERAPY

1. Balliet R, Shinn J, Bach-Y-Rita P. Facial paralysis rehabilitation: retraining selective muscle control. Int Rehabil Med 1982;4:67–74.

2. Henklemann T. Physical therapy in neuro muscular rehabilitation. In: May M, Schaitkin BM, editors. The facial nerve. New York: Thieme; 2000. p. 301–17.

3. Ross BG, Fradet G, Nedzelski JM. Development of a sensitive clinical facial grading system. Otolaryngol Head Neck Surg 1996;114:380–6.

4. Diels HJ. A new concept in non-surgical facial nerve rehabilitation. In: Myers EN, Bluestone CD, Brackmann DE, et al, editors. Advances in otolaryngology—head and neck surgery, vol. 9. Chicago Moseby Yearbook; 1995. p. 289.

5. Mehta RP, Hadlock TA. Botulinum toxin and quality of life in patients with facial paralysis. Arch Facial Plast Surg 2008;10:84–7.

6. Teixeira LJ, Soares BG, Vieira VP, et al. Physical therapy for Bells palsy (idiopathic facial paralysis). Cochrane Database Syst Rev 2008;3:CD006283.

7. Lai D, Hetzler LT, Sharma N, et al. Electrical stimulation facilitates rat facial nerve recovery from a crush injury. Otolaryngol Head Neck Surg 2008;1:68–73.

8. Manikandan N. Effective fisual neuromuscular reeducation on facial symmetry in patients with Bell's Palsy: a randomized control trial. Clin Rehabil 2007;4:338–43.

9. Hadlock TA, Greenfield LJ, Wernick-Robinson M, et al. Mutimodality approach to management of the paralyzed face. Laryngoscope 2006;116:1385–9.

PREOPERATIVE ASSESSMENT TOOLS

10. Moe KS, Kao CH. Precaruncular medial canthopexy. Arch Facial Plast Surg 2005;7:244–50.
11. May M, Schaitkin BM. The facial nerve. In: May M, Schaitkin BM, editors. Reporting recovery of facial function. 2nd edition. New York: Thieme Medical Publishers; 2000. p. 275–94.
12. Morel-Fatio D, Lalardie JP. Palliative surgical treatment of facial paralysis: the Palpebral Spring. Plast Reconstr Surg 1964;33:446–56.
13. Levine RE, Shapiro JP. Reanimation of the paralyzed eyelid with the enhanced palpebral spring or the gold weight: modern replacements for tarsorrhaphy. Facial Plast Surg 2000;16:325–36.
14. Rubin LP. Anatomy of a smile. In: Rubin LP, editor. The paralyzed face. St Louis (MO): Mosby; 1991.

ASSESSMENT OF RESULTS OF FACIAL PARALYSIS

15. Reporting recovery of facial function. In: Schaitkin BM, May M, editors. The Facial Nerve May's Second Edition. New York: Thieme; 2000.
16. Vrabec JT, Backous DD, Djalilian HR, et al. Facial Nerve Grading System 2.0. Otolaryngol Head Neck Surg 2009;4:445–50.
17. Ross BG, Fradet G, Nedzelski JM. Development of a sensitive clinical facial grading system. Otolaryngol Head Neck Surg 1996;114:380–6.
18. Yamamoto Y, Sekido M, Furukawa H, et al. Surgical rehabilitation of reversible facial palsy: facial–hypoglossal network system based on neural signal augmentation/neural supercharge concept. J Plast Reconstr Aesthet Surg 2007; 60(3):223–31.

"DISCUSS THE USE OF END-TO-SIDE ANASTOMOSIS (VITERBO CONCEPT OF SOMETHING FOR NOTHING). SHOULD IT BE USED; WHY OR WHY NOT?"

19. Viterbo F, Trindaade JC, Hoshino K, et al. Lateroterminal neurorrhaphy without removal of the epineural sheath: experimental study in rats. Rev Paul Med 1992;110:267–75.
20. Frey M, Giovanoli P, Michaelidou M. Functional upgrading of partially recovered facial palsy by cross-face nerve grafting with distal end-to-side neurorrhaphy. Plast Reconstr Surg 2006;117(2): 597–608.
21. Brenner MJ, Dvali L, Hunter DA, et al. Motor neuron regeneration through end-to-side repairs is a function of donor nerve axotomy. Plast Reconstr Surg 2007;120(1):215–23.

"WHAT IS YOUR PREFERRED METHOD FOR TEMPORALIS MUSCLE TRANSPOSITION AND WHY? ARE THERE ANY TRICKS TO IMPROVING THE RESULTS?"

22. Croxson GR, Qunn MJ, Coulson SE. Temporalis muscle transfer for facial paralysis: a further refinement. Facial Plast Surg 2000;16(4):351–6.
23. Byrne PJ, Kim M, Boahene K, et al. The Temporalis tendon transfer as part of a comprehensive approach to facial reanimation. Arch Facial Plast Surg 2007;9(4):234–41.
24. Gillies H. Experiences with Fascia Lata Grafts in the Operative Treatment of Facial Paralysis. Proc R Soc Med 1934;27(10):1372–82.
25. McLaughlin CR. Surgical support in permanent facial paralysis. Plast Reconstr Surg 1953;11(4): 302–14.
26. Boahene KD, Farrag TY, Ishii L, et al. Minimally invasive temporalis tendon transposition. Arch Facial Plast Surg 2011;13(1):8–13.
27. Hadlock TA, Greenfield LJ, Wernick-Robinso M, et al. Mutimodality approach to management of the paralyzed face. Laryngoscope 2006;116: 1385–9.

Index

Note: Page numbers of article titles are in **boldface** type.

A

Facial Plast Surg Clin N Am 20 (2012) 403–414
http://dx.doi.org/10.1016/S1064-7406(12)00069-7

Printed and bound by CPI Group (UK) Ltd, Croydon, CR0 4YY

03/10/2024

01040359-0009